Contemporary Diagnosis
and Management of

The Post-MI Patient®

Ezra A. Amsterdam, MD
Professor of Medicine
Director, Cardiac Care Unit
Division of Cardiovascular Medicine
Department of Internal Medicine
University of California, Davis, School of
Medicine and Medical Center, Sacramento

and

Philip R. Liebson, MD
Professor of Medicine and Preventive Medicine
Associate Director, Section of Cardiology
Rush Medical College
Rush-Presbyterian-St Luke's Medical Center
Chicago, Illinois

Published by Handbooks in Health Care Co.,
Newtown, Pennsylvania, USA

Acknowledgments

This volume is dedicated to our families, patients, and students.

The authors express their appreciation for the skilled administrative efforts of Shirl Fischer and for the support of Marvin Anzel, Publisher; Matthew Corso, Vice President, Communications; and Robin Henry, Senior Editor, of Handbooks in Health Care.

International Standard Book Number: 1-931981-54-X

Library of Congress Catalog Card Number: 2005932018

Second Edition

Table of Contents

This book has been prepared and is presented as a service to the medical community. The information provided reflects the knowledge, experience, and personal opinions of the authors, Ezra A. Amsterdam, MD, Professor of Medicine, Director, Cardiac Care Unit, Division of Cardiovascular Medicine, Department of Internal Medicine, University of California, Davis, School of Medicine and Medical Center, Sacramento, California, and Philip R. Liebson, MD, Professor of Medicine and Preventive Medicine, Associate Director, Section of Cardiology, Rush Medical College, Rush-Presbyterian-St. Luke's Medical Center, Chicago, Illinois.

This book is not intended to replace or to be used as a substitute for the complete prescribing information prepared by each manufacturer for each drug. Because of possible variations in drug indications, in dosage information, in newly described toxicities, in drug/drug interactions, and in other items of importance, reference to such complete prescribing information is definitely recommended before any of the drugs discussed are used or prescribed.

Preface

Despite remarkable progress in the treatment of cardiovascular disease and a continuing decrease in mortality, heart disease remains the leading cause of death in the United States. Coronary heart disease (CHD), the primary etiology of this medical, social, and economic crisis, accounts for more than 500,000 deaths each year. Acute myocardial infarction (MI), one of the most dramatic and devastating manifestations of CHD, occurs in more than 1 million Americans each year, and it is fatal in one third of victims. Thus, each year, more than 600,000 patients join the ranks of survivors of acute MI, indicating the magnitude of this problem, which includes millions of patients. Moreover, one result of current therapeutic success is a continuing increase in the number of these patients. In addition to a high rate of disability, they are at increased risk for recurrent fatal and nonfatal coronary events. Although recent clinical trials of post-MI therapy have demonstrated major strides in reducing post-MI morbidity and mortality, a continuing paradox in current practice is the lack of consistent application of these findings to direct patient care. This dilemma is particularly obvious in the underuse of cardioprotective pharmacologic and nondrug treatment, a phenomenon referred to as the 'knowledge-practice gap.' Therefore, the goal of this handbook is promotion of optimal management of survivors of acute MI based on rational application of contemporary scientific knowledge.

We strongly advocate evidence-based medicine and the use of current guidelines, such as those of the American College of Cardiology/American Heart Association. This approach comprises the scientific basis of medical practice. The art of medicine is application of this science to the *individual* patient. Key and complementary elements in this process are knowledge and judgment. To this end, this handbook is divided into chapters on the pathophysiology of ischemic heart disease, particularly acute MI; coronary risk factors and their management; determinants of early and late post-MI prognosis; methods of post-MI risk stratification and indications for invasive studies; indications for and results of cardioprotective medical therapy; psychological issues in the post-MI patient; and resumption of activity during inpatient convalescence and following hospital discharge. Each chapter is extensively illustrated with figures and tables from major classic and contemporary studies, which afford a detailed bibliography of the subject. These studies are listed at the end of each chapter. Appendixes provide relevant guidelines of the American College of Cardiology and American Heart Association, selected Web sites for further information, and a short list of texts for reference. Throughout, we emphasize and recommend the value and limitations of diagnostic techniques and therapeutic choices, based on current trials. Our focus is on patients with uncomplicated MI or those who have been stabilized after a complicated MI. The complications of acute MI and their management are covered in excellent current texts on these subjects.

Comprehensive management of the post-MI patient includes many forms of testing and treatment. Our challenge is to understand the bases of these approaches, their indications, and the results of their application in the unique context presented by each patient. If this book contributes to increased awareness of these issues, leading to enhanced management of post-MI patients, we will have realized our objective.

Chapter 1

Myocardial Infarction in the Spectrum of Coronary Artery Disease

Despite major advances in the treatment and prevention of coronary heart disease (CHD) that have reduced its incidence during the past 4 decades, CHD due to coronary atherosclerosis continues to surpass all other causes of mortality in industrialized societies. The grim toll of CHD in human and economic terms in the United States is reflected by more than 500,000 deaths each year and by a cost of more than $20 billion in medical care for the 14 million patients with one or more forms of the disease. The annual incidence of acute myocardial infarction (MI) in the United States is estimated at 1.2 million to 1.5 million cases, of which more than one third are fatal before the victim reaches a hospital. However, of those who are hospitalized, survival has steadily risen from 70% 30 years ago to approximately 90% today. Thus, almost 1 million patients stricken with acute MI survive and are discharged from the hospital annually. This group, which is at high risk for recurrent events, has benefited from recent therapeutic innovations, including cardioprotective drugs, revascularization therapy, and lifestyle changes. These innovations have significantly improved long-term prognosis after acute MI.

Optimal management of the post-MI patient requires (1) a systematic approach to assess the risk for recurrent coronary events; and (2) appropriate application of the growing number of therapeutic options that have had a favorable effect on prognosis. The foundation of this strategy is an understanding of current concepts of the pathophysiology of CHD and its complications.

The Spectrum of Coronary Heart Disease

Coronary artery disease produces a number of clinical syndromes that make up the spectrum of CHD, of which acute MI is the most frequent initial manifestation (Table 1-1). The other major clinical presentations of CHD are angina pectoris and sudden death. Estimates vary, but current data suggest that acute MI is the initial expression of CHD in 40% to 50% of patients. Angina pectoris is the first indication of the disease in 30% to 40% of patients; sudden death (defined as death within 1 hour of onset of symptoms) is the presenting finding in 10% to 20% of CHD victims.

Additional complications of CHD include unstable angina (which is occasionally CHD's first manifestation), arrhythmias, and congestive heart failure (CHF). The latter is usually related to extensive loss of myocardium from one or more MIs. A striking message of these statistics is that the initial presentation of CHD in most patients is a human catastrophe: MI or sudden death. Furthermore, angina pectoris is the first clinical finding in a minority of patients. Thus, primary prevention on a wide scale is obviously needed to achieve a major reduction in the burden of CHD.

Traditional Classification

The most common symptom of myocardial ischemia is chest discomfort. When this symptom is severe and prolonged (ie, >20 minutes), acute MI or unstable angina should be considered. The diagnosis of MI continues to be based on at least two of the following three major clinical findings: compatible symptoms (usually typical chest discomfort), evolution of pathologic Q waves on electrocardiogram (ECG), and characteristic changes in serum markers of cardiac injury. MI was traditionally categorized as transmural or nontransmural (or subendocardial), based on the presence or absence, respectively, of pathologic Q waves on ECG. In the absence of ECG evolution of pathologic Q waves (40 msec duration), elevations of serum markers of cardiac injury were required for the diagnosis of nontransmural MI, while unstable angina was indicated if there was no elevation of serum markers. Although both nontransmural MI and unstable angina were commonly associated with ischemic electrocardiographic abnormalities, such as horizontal ST depression and/or symmetrical, deep T-wave inversion (>3 mm), ECG alterations have not been required for diagnosis of these syndromes.

Contemporary Classification

Although it does not differ fundamentally from the traditional categories, recent classification of the acute ischemic manifestations of CHD is more closely based on recent understanding of the underlying pathophysiology, described in detail below. According to current concepts, acute myocardial ischemia/infarction is viewed as a continuum from unstable angina to non-Q-wave MI and Q-wave MI. These disorders are collectively considered the acute coronary syndromes (ACS). Clinicians now recognize the limitations of former classifications relating the ECG to MI pathology in that Q-wave MI is not consistently transmural. Moreover, the recent development of increasingly sensitive serum markers of cardiac injury, such as the troponins, has blurred the distinction between non-Q-wave MI and unstable angina.

All ACS are characterized by prolonged chest pain compatible with myocardial ischemia/infarction. The diagnosis of each is based on subsequent ECG alterations and serum marker data. Q-wave MI is recognized in its early stages by ST-segment elevation and is, therefore, termed STEMI. Non-Q-wave MI is referred to as non-STEMI, or NSTEMI ACS. Both STEMI and NSTEMI are, by definition, associated with elevation of serum markers of myocardial injury. Absence of the latter in NSTEMI defines unstable angina. These relationships are depicted in Figure 1-1. Refined diagnostic methods for detecting cardiac injury have confirmed the continuous nature of myocardial ischemia/infarction, resulting in the concept of minimal myocardial damage for borderline elevations of the troponins, now the most sensitive and specific indicators of myocardial injury. The arbitrary classification of unstable angina and non-Q-wave MI, which are part of the continuum of CHD, is also reflected by the direct correlation of mortality with the degree of elevation of the troponins in NSTEMI.

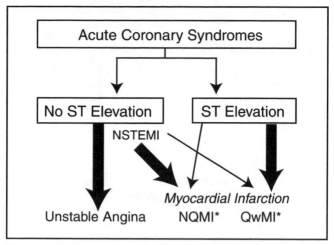

Figure 1-1: Nomenclature of acute coronary syndromes (ACS). Patients with ischemic discomfort may present with or without ST-segment elevation (STE) on the electrocardiogram (ECG). Most patients with STE (large arrows) ultimately develop a Q-wave acute myocardial infarction (MI) (QwMI), whereas a minority (small arrows) develop a non-Q-wave acute MI (NQMI). Patients who present without STE are experiencing either unstable angina (UA) or a non-ST-elevation MI (NSTEMI). The distinction between these two diagnoses is ultimately made based on the presence or absence of a cardiac marker detected in the blood. Most patients with NSTEMI do not evolve a Q wave on the 12-lead ECG and are subsequently referred to as having sustained a NQMI; only a minority of NSTEMI patients develop a Q wave and are later diagnosed as having QwMI. Not shown is Prinzmetal's angina, which presents with transient chest pain and STE but rarely MI. The spectrum of clinical conditions that ranges from UA to NQMI and QwMI is referred to as ACS.

*Elevation of cardiac injury marker.

Reproduced with permission from Antman EM, Braunwald E: Acute myocardial infarction. In: Braunwald E, ed. *Heart Disease: A Textbook of Cardiovascular Medicine,* 5th ed, vol 2. Philadelphia, PA, WB Saunders, 1997, pp 1184-1288.

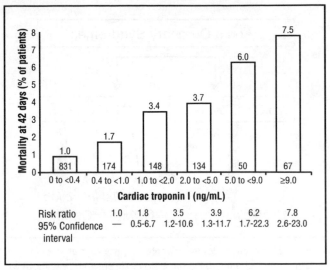

Figure 1-2: Relationship between cardiac troponin I levels and risk of mortality in patients with acute coronary syndromes. Reproduced with permission from Antman et al, *N Engl J Med* 1996;335:1342-1349.

This is indicated in Figure 1-2, which demonstrates that mortality begins to rise with even small elevations of the troponins.

Pathogenesis of Acute Myocardial Infarction

Plaque Rupture

Myocardial infarction is the irreversible necrosis of cardiac muscle that results from an inadequate oxygen supply caused by the interruption of coronary blood flow to the myocardium. Infarction can involve any chamber of the heart, but it most frequently occurs in the left ventricle because of this ventricle's high oxygen requirements, which considerably surpass those of the other cardiac chambers. In approximately 90% of patients with acute

MI, this impairment of blood supply is the result of acute thrombotic obstruction of a coronary artery. Recent studies indicate that coronary thrombosis is initiated by rupture of an atherosclerotic plaque that induces a cascade of vasculo-occlusive mechanisms. Plaque rupture exposes the thrombogenic subendothelial collagen matrix, which induces local aggregation of platelets, promoting superimposition of fibrin deposition to form a thrombus at the site of ulceration. Activated platelets release factors, such as thromboxane A_2 and serotonin, that provoke vasospasm and augment platelet activity, inducing further aggregation, hemostasis, and thrombogenesis. These pathogenic mechanisms overwhelm endogenous vasodilator and antithrombotic factors, such as prostacyclin and tissue plasminogen activator, whose production by diseased endothelium is inadequate to offset the intense thrombotic activity initiated by plaque rupture.

Evolution and Extent of Myocardial Infarction

Coronary thrombosis is usually acute but may evolve over minutes or many hours, depending on the degree of imbalance between prothrombotic and antithrombotic mechanisms at the site of plaque rupture. However, for myocardial necrosis to occur, the imbalance between myocardial oxygen requirements and oxygen supply must be severe and prolonged. Infarction is a dynamic process, with myocardial necrosis usually progressing to completion in a jeopardized region over 6 to 8 hours after interruption of blood supply (Figure 1-3). The interval varies, depending on the determinants of myocardial oxygen demand (heart rate, blood pressure, contractility, ventricular volume) and oxygen supply (collateral coronary arteries, arterial Po_2, diastolic time interval, diastolic coronary perfusion gradient) during the coronary occlusive process. An understanding of these factors provides the basis for contemporary management of acute MI, the primary goal of which is limiting the extent of myocardial injury and

13

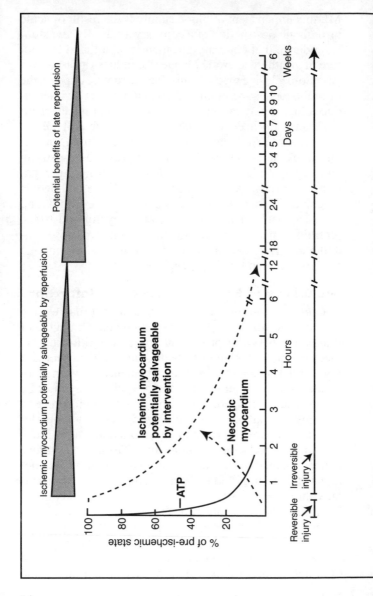

	Sarcolemmal disruption: mitochondrial amorphous densities					
Electron microscopy	Glycogen depletion; mitochondrial swelling; relaxation of myofibrils					
Histochemistry				← TTC staining defect →		
Light microscopy	Waviness of fibers at border	Beginning coagulation necrosis; edema; focal hemorrhage; beginning neutrophilic infiltrate	Continuing coagulation necrosis; pallor (shrunken nuclei and eosinophilic cytoplasm); myosite contraction bands	Coagulation necrosis with loss of nuclei and striations; neutrophilic infiltrate	Disintegration of myofibers and phagocytosis by macrophages	Completion of phagocytosis; prominent granulation tissue with neovascularization and fibrovascular reaction	Mature fibrous scar
Gross changes			Pallor	Pallor, sometimes hyperemia; yellowing at periphery	Hyperemic border, central yellow-brown softening	Maximally yellow and soft vascularized edges; red-brown and depressed	

Figure 1-3: Temporal sequence of early biochemical, ultrastructural, histochemical, and histological findings after onset of myocardial infarction. At the top of the figure, schematically shown, are the time frames for early and late reperfusion of the myocardium supplied by an occluded coronary artery. For approximately one half hour following the onset of even the most severe ischemia, myocardial injury is potentially reversible; after that, there is progressive loss of viability that is complete by 6 to 12 hours. The benefits of reperfusion (early and late) are greatest when it is achieved early, with progressively smaller benefits occurring as reperfusion is delayed. Reproduced with permission from Gersh BJ, Braunwald E, Bonow RO: Chronic coronary artery disease. In: Braunwald E, ed. *Heart Disease: A Textbook of Cardiovascular Medicine*, 5th ed, vol 2. Philadelphia, PA, WB Saunders, 1997, pp 1184-1288.

Figure 1-4: Diagram demonstrating characteristics of 'vulnerable' and 'stable' atherosclerotic plaques. The vulnerable plaque usually has a substantial lipid core and a thin fibrous cap separating the thrombogenic macrophages (bearing tissue factor) from the blood. At sites of lesion disruption, smooth muscle cells (SMCs) are often activated. In contrast, the stable plaque has a thick fibrous cap protecting the lipid core from contact with the blood. Clinical data suggest that stable plaques more often show luminal narrowing detectable by angiography than do vulnerable plaques. Reproduced with permission from Libby, *Circulation* 1995;91:2844-2850.

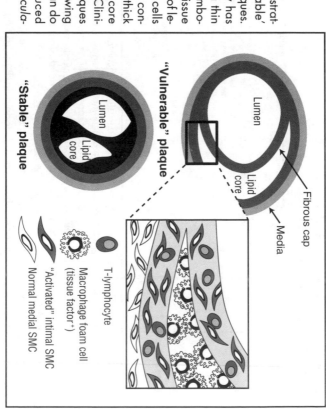

thereby reducing MI size. The importance of this objective is reflected by the fact that MI size, or the amount of myocardial damage, is one of the primary determinants, if not *the* primary determinant, of short-term and long-term clinical outcome.

Vulnerable and Stable Plaques

Knowledge of the pathophysiology of acute MI indicates why this drastic clinical event is so often the initial manifestation of CHD without prior warning by a less severe clinical syndrome such as stable angina. According to current concepts, the plaque that ulcerates and sets in motion the cascade of thrombogenesis and coronary occlusion possesses a thin fibrous cap and a large lipid pool (Figure 1-4). It is also the site of multiple mediators of inflammation that promote ulceration and rupture of the fibrous cap. Because it is prone to rupture, it is referred to as a vulnerable plaque. In contrast, a stable plaque is characterized by a thick fibrous cap and a relatively small lipid pool, has little evidence of inflammatory activity, and is, thus, less subject to ulceration with consequent coronary thrombosis. The vulnerable plaque is typically noncritical in terms of the degree of coronary stenosis it produces in its quiescent state, which is usually less than 70% reduction of lumen diameter. Symptoms of myocardial ischemia do not usually occur with this degree of stenosis because it does not significantly impair coronary blood flow at rest or augmentation with stress. Reduction of the latter (coronary blood flow reserve) is associated with stenoses greater than 70%, while impairment of resting coronary flow occurs when lumen diameter is reduced by >90%. These relationships are depicted in Figure 1-5. Thus, most vulnerable plaques are clinically 'silent' until rupture and thrombosis occur. These findings further emphasize the importance of prevention of atherosclerosis in combating CHD. Plaque structure is not static and may shift

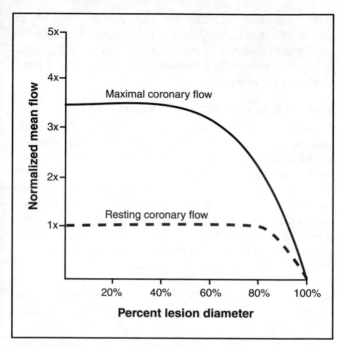

Figure 1-5: Resting and maximal coronary blood flow are affected by the magnitude of proximal arterial stenosis (percent lesion diameter). The dotted line indicates resting blood flow, and the solid line represents maximal blood flow (ie, when there is a full dilatation of the distal resistance vessels). Compromise of maximal blood flow is evident when the proximal stenosis reduces the coronary lumen diameter by more than ~70%. Resting flow may be compromised if the stenosis exceeds ~90%. Reproduced with permission from Gould et al, *Am J Cardiol* 1974;34:50.

between the more stable and the relatively vulnerable states during the course of a patient's disease, depending on the influence of risk factors, therapy, and hemodynamic alterations.

Pathophysiology of the Acute Coronary Syndromes

The degree of thrombotic coronary obstruction typically determines which form of ACS ensues after plaque ulceration and coronary thrombosis. A totally occlusive thrombus completely interrupts regional myocardial blood flow, resulting in STEMI and, usually, substantial myocardial necrosis. A partially occlusive thrombus produces incomplete reduction of coronary blood flow and severe myocardial ischemia, resulting in either NSTEMI (elevation of serum markers) or unstable angina (no elevation of serum markers). The degree of elevation of serum markers in ACS generally, but not always, correlates with the extent of myocardial damage and, therefore, with morbidity and mortality (Figure 1-2).

As previously stated, there is a general correlation between the pathogenesis of MI and the extent of myocardial damage. Because NSTEMI usually involves less cardiac muscle loss than STEMI, mortality and other serious complications, such as cardiogenic shock, CHF, and serious arrhythmias, are less frequent during the initial hospitalization in the former than the latter. However, in some cases, NSTEMI may result in extensive damage and STEMI may be associated with lesser injury. Furthermore, recurrent events are common with NSTEMI. Infarct size is also related to additional factors, such as the specific 'culprit' coronary artery, the site of vessel occlusion, presence of collateral coronary arteries, and (as indicated above) the hemodynamic factors influencing myocardial oxygen demand and supply during the evolution of the infarction. Thus, because the left anterior descending coronary artery usually supplies the largest area of myocardium, its occlusion generally results in more extensive damage than does occlusion of the right or left circumflex artery. Proximal coronary occlusion is associated with greater injury than distal occlusion; collateral coronaries can limit the extent of infarction, as can factors favoring reduced myocardial oxygen demand (eg, lower heart rate and blood pressure).

Nonatherosclerotic Causes of Myocardial Infarction

Although uncommon, MI can occur in the absence of coronary atherosclerosis. Nonatherosclerotic etiologies include coronary vasospasm, coronary emboli, vasculitis, congenital anomalies, trauma, and excessive myocardial oxygen demand in the presence of normal coronary arteries. The latter derangement can occur with cocaine abuse (vasospasm as well as hypertension and tachycardia), severe aortic stenosis, and hypertrophic obstructive cardiomyopathy. Cocaine and other drugs of abuse, such as methamphetamines, should be considered in young patients presenting with ACS, particularly those with few or no cardiovascular risk factors. These agents can be screened for by urine toxicology studies on admission.

Diagnosis of Acute Myocardial Infarction

Recent guidelines of the American College of Cardiology and the American Heart Association provide recommendations for management of ACS according to current standards of care, based on clinical evidence of efficacy. As stated earlier, diagnosis of acute MI continues to be based on at least two of three of the following factors:

(1) Compatible symptoms, which usually consist of pressure-like retrosternal discomfort. Other presentations, such as dyspnea and mental status changes, are not uncommon, particularly in women and the elderly, in whom atypical symptoms are relatively common.

(2) Electrocardiogram alterations of injury consisting of ST-segment elevation (Figure 1-6), which may or may not evolve with the development of pathologic Q waves. This depends on the timeliness of therapy, particularly coronary reperfusion. Other ECG changes, such as ST-segment depression and T-wave inversion, are consistent

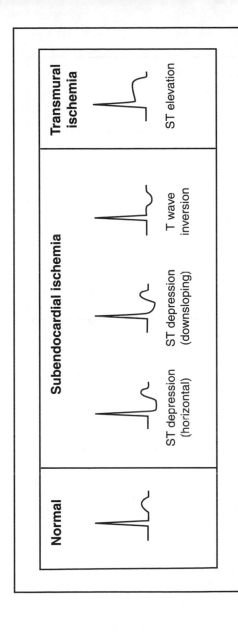

Figure 1-6: Common transient electrocardiogram abnormalities during ischemia. Subendocardial ischemia results in ST-segment depressions and/or T-wave flattening or inversions. Severe transient transmural ischemia can result in ST-segment elevations, similar to the early changes in acute myocardial infarction. When transient ischemia resolves, so do the electrocardiographic changes. Reproduced with permission from Sabatine MS, O'Gara PT, Lilly LS: Ischemic heart disease. In: Lilly LS, ed. *Pathophysiology of Heart Disease*, 2nd ed. Baltimore, MD, Lippincott Williams & Wilkins, 1998, p 134.

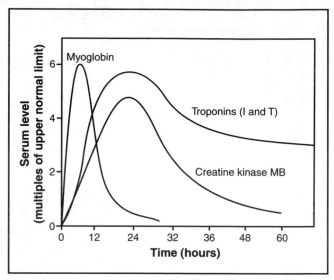

Figure 1-7: Patterns of evolution of serum markers after onset of myocardial necrosis. Reproduced with permission from Amsterdam et al, *Cardiol Rev* 1999;7:17-26.

with ischemia but have many other possible causes. They can provide further evidence of ACS in patients with compatible clinical presentations.

(3) Evolution of serum markers of cardiac injury (Figure 1-7), which is now based primarily on troponin I or T because of their superior sensitivity and specificity for detecting infarction. Because of the prolonged elevation of the troponins (7 to 14 days) after MI, measurement of the MB fraction of creatine kinase remains useful for identifying early reinfarction.

Management of Acute Myocardial Infarction

The initial management of acute MI entails a comprehensive approach with the goals of early relief of symptoms and prevention of mortality and morbidity related to the acute event. In survivors of MI, the objectives are long-term prevention of recurrent events and restoration of optimal functional status. Modern management of acute MI is based on rapid diagnosis and early institution of therapy. Current recommendations include obtaining and interpreting an ECG within 10 minutes in all adults presenting to the emergency department with symptoms consistent with ACS, most typically chest discomfort.

ST-elevation Myocardial Infarction

For patients with ST-segment elevation and no contraindications, pharmacologic reperfusion therapy should be initiated within 30 minutes of presentation. Other medications administered at initial presentation include oxygen and aspirin. Analgesia should be used if indicated. In the absence of contraindications, patients should receive a nitrate and a β-blocker. An angiotensin-converting enzyme (ACE) inhibitor should be added early (first or second day). Use of this battery of medications assumes no contraindications to these agents, which may include low blood pressure (nitrate, β-blocker, ACE inhibitor) or low heart rate (β-blocker). Based on recent data, one of the statins can also be administered early in the course of infarction to initiate the benefits of lipid lowering early and to capitalize on statins' potential anti-inflammatory actions during the acute phase of MI. In hospitals with cardiac catheterization laboratories and expertise in acute coronary intervention, the preferred method for coronary reperfusion is primary angioplasty with stent placement. Coronary stent placement also involves short-term administration of a platelet glycoprotein IIB/IIIA inhibitor for optimal stent patency. Reduction of mortality and morbidity of 20% to 35% in patients with acute MI has been demonstrated with the use of reperfusion therapy (pharmacologic or angioplasty), aspirin, β-blockers, and ACE inhibitors. These agents attenuate mortality and morbidity by a variety of mechanisms, which include one or more of the following pathologic processes: thrombosis, ischemia, arrhythmias, and left ventricular remodeling.

Non-ST-elevation Acute Coronary Syndromes

If the patient presenting with chest pain has NSTEMI ACS, based on cardiac serum markers and/or ECG changes, initial therapy includes aspirin, heparin, nitrates, and a β-blocker. Recent findings indicate that clopidogrel (Plavix®) reduces combined ischemic events in NSTEMI ACS and, therefore, should be added to initial treatment. An ACE inhibitor and a statin are also important components of early therapy. If this management fails to alleviate symptoms and/or ischemia, more intensive therapy involves addition of a platelet IIB/IIIA inhibitor and/or coronary intervention. It should be stated that in most patients with NSTEMI ACS, intensive medical therapy provides appropriate initial management.

Post-acute Hospital Phase

Overall survival in patients reaching the hospital with acute MI is approximately 90%. However, this varies widely and may be close to 100% in the lowest-risk patients (young patients with small, uncomplicated MIs) and <50% in the highest-risk group (elderly patients with large, complicated MIs). Similarly, long-term prognosis varies considerably in those patients surviving to leave the hospital, depending on multiple factors that influence prognosis and the use of the increasing array of cardioprotective therapy. Subsequent chapters will consider the fundamental questions of assessment of prognosis and selection of therapy in survivors of acute MI.

Suggested Readings

Amsterdam EA, Lewis WR, Yadlapalli S: Evaluation of low-risk patients with chest pain in the emergency department: value and limitations of recent methods. *Cardiol Rev* 1999;7:17-26.

Antman EM, Braunwald EM: Acute myocardial infarction. In: Braunwald E, ed. *Heart Disease: A Textbook of Cardiovascular Medicine*. 5th ed, vol 2. Philadelphia, PA, WB Saunders Co, 1997, pp 1184-1288.

Antman EM, Tanasijevic MJ, Thompson B, et al: Cardiac-specific troponin I levels to predict the risk of mortality in patients with acute coronary syndromes. *N Engl J Med* 1996;335:1342-1349.

Braunwald E, Antman EM, Beasley JW, et al: ACC/AHA 2002 guideline update for the management of patients with unstable angina and non-ST-segment elevation myocardial infarction: a report of the American College of Cardiology/American Heart Association Task Force on Practice Guidelines (Committee on the Management of Patients With Unstable Angina). *J Am Coll Cardiol* 2002;40:1366-1374. Available at: http://www.acc.org/clinical/guidelines/unstable/unstable.pdf. Accessed on May 16, 2003.

Gould KL, Lipscomb K: Effects of coronary stenoses on coronary flow reserve and resistance. *Am J Cardiol* 1974;34:48-55.

Libby P: Molecular bases of the acute coronary syndromes. *Circulation* 1995;91:2844-2850.

Lilly LS, ed: *Pathophysiology of Heart Disease.* 2nd ed. Baltimore, MD, Lippincott Williams & Wilkins, 1998.

Ryan TJ, Antman EM, Brooks NH, et al: ACC/AHA guidelines for the management of patients with acute myocardial infarction: 1999 update: a report of the American College of Cardiology/American Heart Association Task Force on Practice Guidelines (Committee on Management of Acute Myocardial Infarction). Available at: http://www.acc.org. Accessed on May 16, 2003.

Chapter 2

Risk Stratification Following Acute Myocardial Infarction

Evaluation of prognosis by systematic risk stratification after acute myocardial infarction (MI) is fundamental to optimal patient management. It provides an estimate of the probability of long-term survival and recurrent coronary events. It is also essential for the rational selection of patients for coronary angiography and myocardial revascularization. Risk stratification is achieved by a comprehensive evaluation, which entails clinical assessment and objective cardiac tests. This process begins with clinical assessment at the time of the patient's admission and is completed by further testing before, or shortly after, hospital discharge. Patients with complicated MI and clinical instability are candidates for direct coronary angiography and potential myocardial revascularization. This chapter pertains only to clinically stable patients.

The specific goals of prognostic assessment in stable post-MI patients are (1) identification of those who are at high or intermediate risk for recurrent coronary events and who may be candidates for myocardial revascularization and (2) identification of those who are at low risk and do not require invasive intervention and management. It is important to emphasize that all post-MI patients should receive comprehensive secondary prevention, as presented in Chapters 3 through 6. The increasing array of cardio-protective drug therapies and lifestyle changes that con-fer clinical benefit has resulted in a challenge to the clini-cian to practice selectivity in referring patients for post-MI angiography and revascularization. The need for careful patient selection for these procedures is further supported by concerns about improving the cost-effectiveness of medi-cal care. This approach is promoted by attention to current guidelines that are based on scientific evidence. However, it is recognized that any guideline is most appropriately applied as one element in the clinician's decision-making process, which is based on all pertinent factors in each patient's case.

Heterogeneity of Risk in Post-MI Patients

As noted in Chapter 1, patients with coronary heart disease (CHD) make up a heterogeneous population in terms of disease severity and prognosis, especially in those who have survived an acute MI. Although survival following MI has improved in recent decades, post-MI patients remain at increased risk for recurrent coronary events (Figure 2-1). As noted in studies more than 30 years ago, mortality is highest in the early period fol-lowing MI and subsequently decreases to a relatively constant rate at 3 to 6 months. After the first year, the average mortality approaches that of patients with stable angina (~5% per year). However, within the entire post-MI population, the spectrum of risk is very broad, with annual mortality ranging from less than 2% to more than 50%. On the basis of these findings, survivors of MI have generally been classified into high-, intermediate-, and low-risk groups. The high-risk group (10% to >50% an-nual mortality) includes approximately 20% of post-MI patients; intermediate-risk patients (5% to 10% annual mortality) account for approximately 25% of the total; the low-risk group (<5% annual mortality) comprises 40%

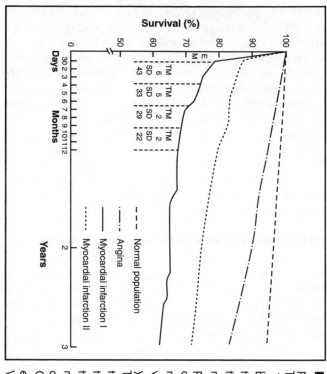

Figure 2-1: Actuarial survival curves for patients with myocardial infarction (MI). The solid line depicts the survival of 1,420 patients with acute MI (I) studied between 1979 and 1984, and the dotted line shows the survival of 1,266 patients (II) followed between sex-matched normal population (dashed line) and patients with angina pectoris (dashed/dotted line). The survival rates in the normal population and angina population were significantly higher at 1, 2, and 3 years. EM = early (30-day) mortality; TM = total mortality (percent) for time interval; SD = sudden death (percent of total mortality) for time intervals during the first year after acute MI. With permission from Henning H: Prognosis of acute myocardial infarction. In: Francis GS, Alpert JS, eds. *Coronary Care*. 2nd ed. Philadelphia, Lippincott Williams & Wilkins, 1995:689-740.

of survivors; and very-low-risk patients (<2% annual mortality) include 15% of the total. This pattern persists into the current era, with contributions from several countervailing mortality trends. Thus, short-term and long-term mortality have fallen because of therapeutic advances and detection of a higher number of small MIs by increasingly sensitive diagnostic methods (eg, serum troponins); by contrast, mortality after MI is considerably elevated in the growing elderly population.

Prognostic Factors

During the past 4 decades, multiple determinants of short-term and long-term prognosis have been identified in survivors of acute MI. Recognition of these variables has been a function of available methodology during any given period. Initial studies of prognosis were based primarily on clinical factors, such as history, physical examination, electrocardiogram (ECG), and radiography. In subsequent investigations, clinical assessment has been complemented by objective data obtained from exercise testing, echocardiography, scintigraphy, and cardiac rhythm monitoring for quantitative evaluation of myocardial ischemia, ventricular function, and arrhythmias. Although the significance of these factors has been influenced by modification of the natural history after acute MI by therapeutic advances, prognostic evaluation remains readily achievable and clinically essential for optimal patient management.

Predictors of short-term and long-term prognosis are available at the time of admission from the history, physical examination, ECG, chest radiograph, and serum cardiac injury markers. Estimates of prognosis from these data can be refined by further evaluation with the aforementioned cardiac tests. This approach applies to patients treated with intravenous thrombolytic agents, although proponents of the 'open artery hypothesis' (see below) advocate definitive angiography to assess coronary

Table 2-1: Peel Prognostic Index

	Score
Sex and age (years):	
Men, 54 or younger	0
55-59	1
60-64	2
65 or older	3
Women, 64 or younger	2
65 or older	3
Previous history:	
Previous cardiac infarct	6
Other cardiovascular diseases or history of exertional dyspnea	3
Angina only	1
No cardiovascular disease	0
Shock:	
Absent	0
Mild–transient at onset	1
Moderate–present on admission but subsiding with rest and sedation	5
Severe–persisting despite rest and sedation	7

Modified with permission from Peel et al, *Br Heart J* 1962;24:745-760.

anatomy in this group. Patients who receive coronary reperfusion therapy by primary angioplasty will already have had coronary angiography and left ventriculography as part of their initial management. Therefore, further prognostic evaluation is usually limited in this group.

	Score
Failure:	
Absent	0
Few basal rales only	1
Any one or more of the following: breathlessness, acute pulmonary edema, orthopnea or dyspnea, gallop rhythm, liver enlargement, edema, or jugular vein distention	4
Electrocardiogram:	
Normal QRS; changes confined to R-T segment or T wave	1
QR complexes	3
QR complexes or bundle-branch block (If no electrocardiogram obtained, mark 4.)	4
Rhythm:	
Sinus	0
Any one or more of the following: atrial fibrillation, flutter; paroxysmal tachycardia; persisting simple tachycardia (110 or more); frequent electrical stimulation, nodal rhythm, or heart block	4

Total patient score = Prognostic index

Result	Died within 28 days	Angina or signs of failure
	Alive on 28th day	Convalescent or symptom free

Estimation of Prognosis
Predictive Models Based on Clinical Factors

The following predictive models, which represent some of the earliest approaches, are based on readily available clinical data.

Peel Prognostic Index

Published more than 40 years ago, this is one of the first systematic methods for predicting outcomes after acute MI, and it clearly demonstrates the value of clinical assessment for predicting both short-term and long-term outcomes (Table 2-1). A score (the prognostic index) is obtained from the weighted values of six clinical factors (age, sex, shock or cardiac failure, cardiac arrhythmia, ECG changes, and history of cardiovascular disease). Weighting is based on the clinical significance of each factor according to the results of clinical assessment at the time of admission. The prognostic index ranges from 1 to 28, with mortality increasing as the score rises, placing patients into one of five categories. After 1 month in the study, the relationship between the initial score and mortality in more than 900 patients was: 1 to 8 (score), <5% (mortality); 9 to 12, 12.5%; 13 to 16, 25%; ≥17, 65%. Thus, for a hypothetical female patient with an acute MI and the following clinical features, the associated scores are: 70 years old (score 3), no prior cardiac history (0), not in shock (0) or cardiac failure (0), pathologic Q waves present (3), and normal sinus rhythm (0). The total score is 6, placing her in the group with less than 5% mortality at 1 month. The initial index was also shown to have long-term prognostic value. For patients who survived to 1 month, 50% survival varied according to initial prognostic index: index 1 to 8, 8 years; 9 to 12, 3 to 4 years; 13 to 16, less than 3 years; ≥17, 2 years. Therefore, if the hypothetical 70-year-old patient is alive at 1 month, she has a 50% chance of surviving 8 years. However, her outlook may be even better because of therapeutic advances that have altered the natural history of CHD since the Peel index was developed.

Norris Prognostic Index

This predictive instrument is based on only four factors, which are obtained from the history and chest radiograph at admission. The score, or prognostic index, is

Table 2-2: Weightings for the Four Factors Selected for Constructing a Coronary Prognostic Index for Long-term Survival

Factor	X	Y
Age (yr) (X_1, Y_1):		
<50	0.2	4.9
50-59	0.4	4.9
60-69	0.6	4.9
70-79	0.8	4.9
80-89	1.0	4.9
Heart size (X_2, Y_2):		
Normal	0	1.7
Doubtfully or definitely enlarged	1	1.7
Lung fields (X_3, Y_3):		
Normal	0	5.1
Pulmonary congestion	0.3	5.1
Interstitial or pulmonary edema	1	5.1
Previous ischemia (X_4, Y_4):		
No previous infarction	0	3.5
Previous infarction	1	3.5

With permission from Norris et al, *Lancet* 1970; 2:485-487.

calculated from the sum of the products (X and Y) of four weighted factors, as shown in Table 2-2. For example, a 55-year-old patient with normal heart size, normal lung fields on chest radiograph, and a history of prior MI has a score of 5.46 ($0.4 \times 4.9 + 0 + 0 + 3.5 = 5.46$). In Figure 2-2, 3-year mortality is depicted in MI survivors who are divided into five groups according to the prog-

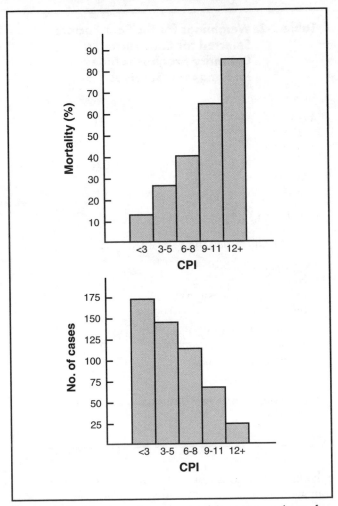

Figure 2-2: Number of patients and 3-year mortality in five groups of patients who had an increasingly poor prognosis as assessed by the coronary prognostic index (CPI) for 3-year survival. Modified with permission from Norris et al, *Lancet* 1970;2:485-487.

nostic index. In this system, the score of the hypothetical patient described above places him in the group with an estimated 3-year mortality of 40%. Norris' original prognostic index, which was devised to predict hospital mortality in MI patients, included two additional factors: ECG location of MI and admission systolic blood pressure. However, these factors were found to be irrelevant to long-term prognosis.

Killip Classification

The physical examination, which provides insight into left ventricular function, is the basis of the familiar Killip classification (Table 2-3). Devised by Killip and Kimball in 1967, this method for predicting outcomes in MI patients is still widely employed for its simplicity and utility. The Killip classes are based on clinical assessment of cardiac function, ranging from absence of heart failure to cardiogenic shock. One-month mortality increases from 5% in class I patients to 80% in class IV patients. Mortality at 1 year remains similarly disparate between the classes.

Multicenter Postinfarction Research Group

Subsequent prognostic models have further refined risk stratification by combining information from clinical and noninvasive assessment. Based on data from almost 900 patients, the Multicenter Postinfarction Research Group reported the risk for mortality during a 2-year interval following MI, in relation to four risk factors (Figure 2-3): previous heart failure, presence of rales, frequent ventricular ectopy, and depressed left ventricular ejection fraction (LVEF). Mortality rose with increasing number of risk factors; the disparity in outcome between patients with no risk factors and those with all four risk factors was 30-fold. Figure 2-3 is a simplified version of the 16 separate survival curves relating mortality and the four risk factors. The shaded areas in the figure represent gradations of risk within the individual risk zones. Note that the highest risk group (four risk

Table 2-3: Hemodynamic Classification of Patients With Acute Myocardial Infarction

Killip Class	Criteria
I	No CHF
II	Basilar rales
III	Pulmonary edema
IV	Shock

CHF = congestive heart failure

* In myocardial infarction patients

** 1-year mortality was not included in the original article and is based on the authors' independent estimates.

Table 2-4: Risk-factor Profile Associated With Low (0.6%) 1-Year Mortality Following Acute Myocardial Infarction

Prior MI	LVEF
No	>40%

MI = myocardial infarction, LVEF = left ventricular ejection fraction, PVCs = premature ventricular contractions

factors) included only 2% of patients, and the patients with lowest risk (no risk factors) made up 33% of the total cohort. The most important predictor in this model was the presence of pulmonary rales, indicating the significance of ventricular dysfunction and confirming the prior concept of Killip.

Incidence*	Mortality (1 mo)	Mortality (1 y)**
30%	<5%	10%
60%	15%	15%
7%	30%	30% to 50%
3%	80%	80% to 100%

Adapted from Killip et al, *Am J Cardiol* 1967;20:457-464.

Complex PVCs	Angina	Exercise Test
Absent	No	Negative

From Ahumada, *Am J Med* 1984;76:900-904.

A subsequent review of multiple studies confirmed a favorable post-MI prognosis in patients with a combination of low-risk findings on clinical assessment, measurement of LVEF, rhythm monitoring, and exercise testing. In patients with the risk profile shown in Table 2-4, 1-year mortality was 0.7%.

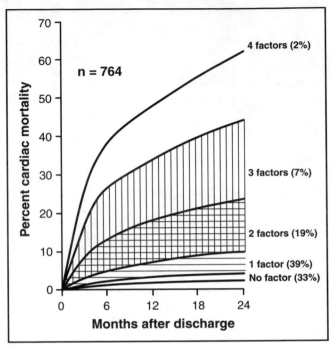

Figure 2-3: Mortality curves after discharge and zones of risk, according to number of risk factors. The risk factors are New York Heart Association functional class II through IV before admission, pulmonary rales, occurrence of 10 or more ventricular ectopic depolarizations per hour, and a radionuclide ejection fraction below 0.40. The variation of risk within each zone reflects the spectrum of relative risk for individual factors. The numbers in the parentheses denote the percentage of the population with the specified number of factors. With permission from *N Engl J Med* 1983;309:331-336.

Other Clinical Factors

Prognosis is related to multiple clinical characteristics not included in the aforementioned scoring systems. Increased prognostic risk is associated with female sex, diabetes, hypertension, obesity in the elderly, conduction defects on ECG, and persistent ST-segment depression (particularly in leads unassociated with new Q waves). These variables likely act through a variety of mechanisms. Female patients with acute MI are generally older; diabetic patients tend to have more extensive coronary artery disease than nondiabetic patients, as well as more widespread vascular disease and target organ damage. Hypertension is associated with left ventricular enlargement and dysfunction.

Electrocardiographic Correlations

Patients can be immediately divided into broad categories of risk based on the ECG alone because it yields critical information on the site and extent of cardiac injury and the culprit coronary artery. The relationship between risk and the initial ECG is clearly depicted in Table 2-5 from the landmark Global Use of Strategies to Open Occluded Arteries in Acute Coronary Syndromes (GUSTO-I) coronary thrombolytic trial. Five ECG categories of acute MI are shown in a cohort of patients who received thrombolysis. Mortality at 30 days and 1 year is highest in extensive anterior MI associated with a conduction disturbance and lowest in isolated inferior MI, in which it is ≤25% of that in the former group. Figure 2-4 demonstrates localization of the infarct artery from the ECG location of the MI. Mortality is typically higher in anterior MI than in inferior MI because the left anterior descending artery normally supplies a greater proportion of the left ventricle than the right or left circumflex coronary artery, and its occlusion results in more extensive damage than that caused by interruption of the latter arteries.

In a study of 911 men hospitalized for non-Q-wave MI or unstable angina, the presence and type of ST-T abnormalities on early ECGs predicted the posthospital clinical course (Figure 2-5). Outcomes were best in the absence of ECG alterations and worst with combined ST elevation and depression. Despite data indicating that non-Q-wave MIs (the former term for non-ST-elevation

Table 2-5: A New Classification of Acute Myocardial Infarction Based on Electrocardiographic Entry Criteria With Angiographic Correlation

Categories

1. Proximal left anterior descending

2. Mid left anterior descending

3. Distal left anterior descending or diagonal

4. Moderate to large inferior (posterior, lateral, right ventricular)

5. Small inferior

*Based on GUSTO-I cohort population in each of the 5 categories, all receiving reperfusion therapy.

MI [NSTEMI]) are smaller than Q-wave MIs (now termed ST-elevation MI [STEMI]), long-term outcomes in this and other studies were comparable in the two populations. Factors correlating with poor long-term outcomes after NSTEMI are high rates of extensive and unstable coronary artery disease and frequent left main

ECG	30-day mortality (%)*	1-year mortality (%)*
ST$\uparrow$ V$_{1-6}$, I, aVL and fascicular or bundle branch block	19.6	25.6
ST$\uparrow$ V$_{1-6}$, I, aVL	9.2	12.4
ST$\uparrow$ V$_1$-V$_4$ or ST$\uparrow$ I, aVL, V$_5$-V$_6$	6.8	10.2
ST$\uparrow$ II, III, aVF and any or all of the following: a. V$_1$, V$_3$R, V$_4$R or b. V$_5$V$_6$ or c. R >S in V$_1$, V$_2$	6.4	8.4
ST$\uparrow$ II, III, aVF only	4.5	6.7

ECG = electrocardiogram, GUSTO-I = Global Use of Strategies to Open Occluded Arteries in Acute Coronary Syndromes

coronary artery involvement. The ECG location of ST-T abnormalities also predicts long-term morbidity and mortality in patients with non-Q-wave MI. In an 18-month follow-up study of 135 patients with non-Q-wave MI, it was found that recurrent MI was significantly more frequent and that survival was significantly lower in pa-

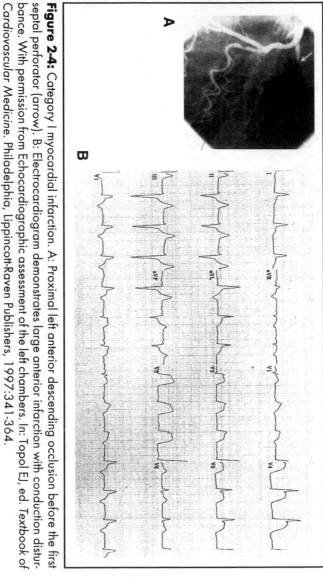

Figure 2-4: Category I myocardial infarction. A: Proximal left anterior descending occlusion before the first septal perforator (arrow). B: Electrocardiogram demonstrates large anterior infarction with conduction disturbance. With permission from Echocardiographic assessment of the left chambers. In: Topol EJ, ed. *Textbook of Cardiovascular Medicine.* Philadelphia, Lippincott-Raven Publishers, 1997:341-364.

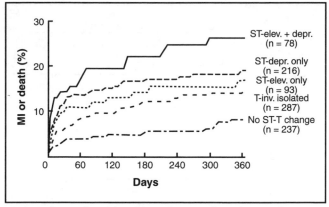

Figure 2-5: Life table of cumulative risk and time of myocardial infarction (MI) or death during 1 year of follow-up with regard to different types of ST-T segment changes in the electrocardiogram (ECG) at rest (n = 911). No ST-T change = normal ECG, n = 237; T-inv. isolated = T-wave inversion without ST-segment change, n = 287; ST-depr. only = ST depression without ST elevation, n = 216; ST-elev. + depr. = combined ST elevation and ST depression, n = 78; ST-elev. only = ST elevation without ST depression, n = 93. With permission from Nyman et al, *J Intern Med* 1993;234:293-301.

tients with anterior ST-T wave changes during the index event than in those with inferior or lateral ST-T alterations (Figures 2-6 and 2-7).

Studies performed during the current era of aggressive management of CHD continue to demonstrate the utility of the ECG in risk-stratifying patients with acute coronary syndromes (ACS). As reported from the Thrombolysis in Myocardial Infarction (TIMI) III Registry of more than 1,400 patients with non-Q-wave MI, those with anterior location of ST-segment deviation had a higher rate of fatal and nonfatal coronary events during the year following admission (Figure 2-8). In this study, isolated

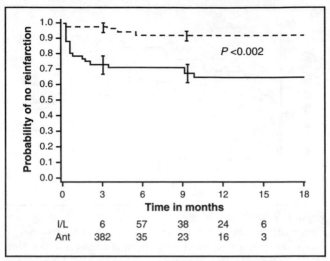

Figure 2-6: Kaplan-Meier probabilities for no reinfarction in patients with anterior non-Q-wave acute myocardial infarction (MI, solid line) and with inferior and/or lateral non-Q-wave acute MI (dotted line). Comparisons of subgroup difference used the method of Cox proportional hazards regression. Ant = anterior; I/L = inferolateral; number indicates total number of patients in each group followed through each time point. With permission from Kao et al, *Am J Cardiol* 1989;64:1236-1242.

T-wave inversion, regardless of location, did not correlate with outcome. The greatest mortality occurred in patients with left bundle branch block, which has also been a high-risk indicator in thrombolytic trials. In this study of patients with non-Q-wave MI, left bundle branch block was the most important ECG predictor of mortality, which was 18% at 1 year, more than double the mortality in patients without this conduction abnormality. It was also observed that cardiac failure was more frequent in this group. The ominous significance of left bundle branch block is most likely related to the occurrence of

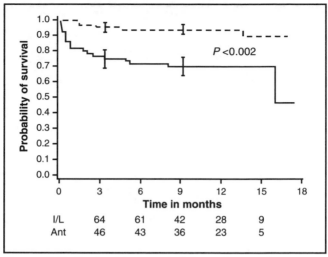

Figure 2-7: Kaplan-Meier probabilities of survival in patients with anterior non-Q-wave acute myocardial infarction (MI, solid line) and with inferior and/or lateral non-Q-wave acute MI (dotted line). Ant = anterior; I/L = inferolateral; number indicates total number of patients in each group followed through each time point. With permission from Kao et al, *Am J Cardiol* 1989;64:1236-1242.

anterior Q-wave MI masked by the conduction abnormality in many of these patients.

In recent studies of patients with non-ST-elevation ACS, ECG evidence of myocardial ischemia has emerged not only as a predictor of high risk, but also as an indicator of which patients will benefit from aggressive therapy that includes early revascularization. Data from the Treat Angina With Aggrastat and Determine Cost of Therapy with an Invasive or Conservative Strategy (TACTICS) trial are shown in Figure 2-9, demonstrating that ST-segment changes identified patients who would benefit from myocardial revascularization.

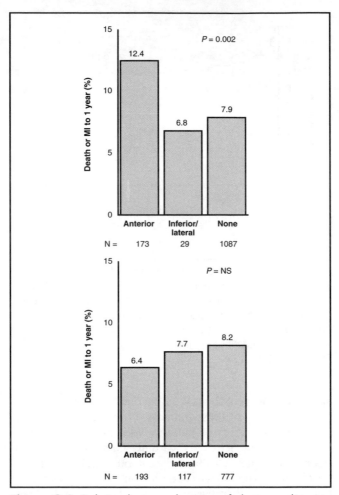

Figure 2-8: Relation between location of electrocardiogram changes and 1-year death or myocardial infarction (MI). Rates are adjusted Kaplan-Meier event rates. Top, ST-segment deviation; bottom, T-wave inversion (includes only those patients with isolated T-wave inversion.) With permission from Cannon et al, *J Am Coll Cardiol* 1997;30:133-140.

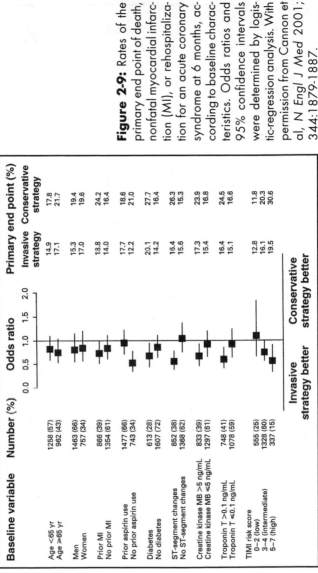

Figure 2-9: Rates of the primary end point of death, nonfatal myocardial infarction (MI), or rehospitalization for an acute coronary syndrome at 6 months, according to baseline characteristics. Odds ratios and 95% confidence intervals were determined by logistic-regression analysis. With permission from Cannon et al, *N Engl J Med* 2001; 344:1879-1887.

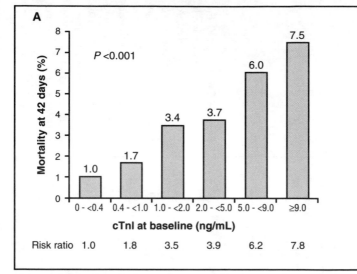

Figure 2-10: Thrombolysis in Myocardial Infarction (TIMI) IIIB. A: A direct relationship was observed between increasing levels of troponin I and a higher 42-day mortality. B: The relationship of positive versus negative troponin I in relation to 42-day mortality in the total group (left) and those with negative creatine kinase

Serum Markers of Cardiac Injury and Inflammation

Release of intracellular macromolecules from injured myocytes affords both diagnostic information and an estimate of the extent of myocardial damage. Because factors such as metabolism, binding, excretion, and 'flushing' from the infarct zone by reperfusion therapy influence the blood level of a cardiac marker, this method is more applicable to populations of MI patients than to individuals. Early studies of this approach revealed that markedly elevated plasma levels ($\geq 2,000$ IU) of creatine kinase (CK) are associated with a poor prognosis and an increased occurrence of left ventricular failure.

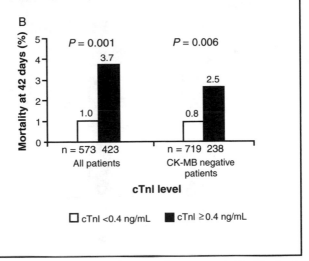

(CK)-MB (right). cTnI = cardiac-specific troponin I. Modified with permission from Cannon C, Braunwald E: Chapter 10. Unstable angina. In: Braunwald E, Zipes D, Libby P, eds. *Heart Disease*. 6th ed. Philadelphia, WB Saunders, 2001, and adapted with permission from Antman et al, *N Engl J Med* 1996;335:1342-1349.

Diagnosis and prognosis based on cardiac injury markers have been improved by the development of reliable assays for the cardiac-specific troponins. As indicated in Figure 2-10A, there is a direct relationship between the blood level of cardiac troponin I and 6-week mortality in patients with non-ST-elevation ACS. Even a small elevation was associated with increased mortality. Further, the troponins have demonstrated superior prognostic value to CK or its MB (myocardial) band. Figure 2-10B, which compares the relationship of CK-MB and troponin I to mortality in patients with non-ST-elevation ACS, indicates that cardiac troponin can discriminate between high- and low-risk patients, even within the group with negative CK-MB values.

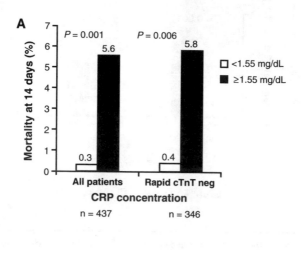

Figure 2-11: Thrombolysis in Myocardial Infarction (TIMI) IIA. A: Relationship of C-reactive protein (CRP) to 14-day mortality in all patients with unstable angina (UA)/non-ST-elevation myocardial infarction (NSTEMI, left) and those with negative baseline troponin T (right). B: Use of both troponin T and CRP to predict mortality. (An 'early positive' rapid bedside troponin T assay [RTnT] was defined as positive in ≤10 minutes.) These data demonstrate that an elevated CRP (the high-sensi-

Current interest in markers of inflammation and CHD risk is considerable. In the TIMI IIA trial of patients with non-ST-elevation ACS, C-reactive protein (CRP) provided prognostic information that was independent of and complementary to that of cardiac troponin T, as shown in Figure 2-11. C-reactive protein identified patients at high risk for short-term mortality even in the group with nega-

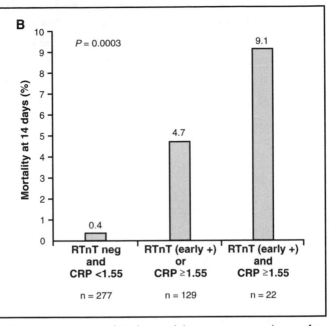

tivity assay was used in this study) is a potent predictor of increased mortality and extends beyond the prognostic information that troponin provides. CRP is a marker of inflammation, whereas the troponins are markers of myocardial necrosis. These data demonstrate the complementary information provided by these two markers in patients with UA/NSTEMI. Early + = early positive; neg = negative. With permission from Morrow et al, *J Am Coll Cardiol* 1998;31:1460-1465.

tive troponin (Figure 2-11A). The complementary predictive value of the two markers is seen in Figure 2-11B. It is emphasized that the use of CRP in this manner requires measurement by the high-sensitivity assay, not the conventional analytic method used in the standard clinical laboratory. Use of the high-sensitivity assay for this marker is designated hs-CRP.

Table 2-6: Hemodynamic Clinical Correlations

Subset	CI	PCP
I, no pulmonary congestion or peripheral hypoperfusion	2.7 ± 0.5	12 ± 7
II, isolated pulmonary congestion	2.3 ± 0.4	23 ± 5
III, isolated peripheral hypoperfusion	1.9 ± 0.4	12 ± 5
IV, both pulmonary congestion and hypoperfusion	1.6 ± 0.6	27 ± 8

CI = cardiac index, PCP = pulmonary capillary pressure

Adapted with permission from Forrester et al, *Am J Cardiol* 1977;39:137-145.

Hemodynamic Data

The extent of myocardial damage and the prognosis can be estimated from measurement of cardiac function. Further, hemodynamic data from bedside right heart catheterization improves the prediction of mortality over that of clinical data. Forrester reported the hemodynamic findings in patients categorized into four clinical subsets based on clinical evidence of pulmonary congestion and hypoperfusion. Left ventricular filling pressure and cardiac output and its derivatives correlated reasonably well with the clinical assessment of hemodynamic impairment (Table 2-6). However, the clinical evaluation failed to recognize the severity of dysfunction in 15% to 20% of patients. Table 2-6 also indicates the marked variation in short-term mortality in the different subsets, reflecting the variable extent of the infarctions. Other studies have reported a fivefold early mortality when left ventricular filling pressure is greater than 20 mm Hg and cardiac index is less than 2.0 L/min/m^2, which usually defines cardiogenic shock and a poor outcome. In patients with left ventricular filling pressure greater than 20 mm Hg, mortality at 2 years is increased twofold.

Noninvasive Cardiac Evaluation

Noninvasive cardiac studies confirmed that post-MI prognosis is closely related to three factors: left ventricular function, myocardial ischemia, and electrical instability. Left ventricular function, which is considered the single most important determinant, is most readily obtained by measuring LVEF by radionuclide ventriculography or echocardiography. Myocardial ischemia and electrical instability are assessed by cardiac stress testing and rhythm monitoring, respectively. The significance of each of these variables is modified by the clinical and demographic factors described in the preceding clinical predictive models.

Left Ventricular Function

Although there may be some restoration of ventricular function by recovery of stunned myocardium after MI, LVEF measured in the peri-MI phase approximates that determined in most patients during the year following discharge. However, detection of viable, ischemic myocardium is an important objective of stress testing. The close, inverse relationship between LVEF and post-MI mortality is a fundamental finding in survivors of MI, as demonstrated in Figure 2-12, based on almost 900 patients from the Multicenter Postinfarction Research Group. One-year mortality is relatively low in patients with normal LVEF and rises sharply as radionuclide ejection fraction falls below 40%; with LVEF less than 30%, mortality increases fivefold. This relationship, based on data primarily from the prethrombolytic period, was confirmed in the thrombolytic era by results from the Gruppo Italiano per lo Studio della Sopravvivenza nell'Infarto Miocardico (GISSI-2) thrombolysis trial obtained by

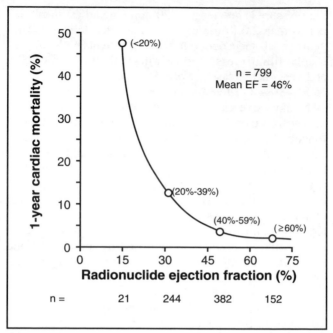

Figure 2-12: Cardiac mortality rate in four categories of radionuclide ejection fraction (EF) determined before discharge (n denotes the number of patients in the total population and in each category). Of 811 patients in whom the EF was recorded, 12 were lost to follow-up during the first year after hospitalization. With permission from *N Engl J Med* 1983;309:331-336.

echocardiography (Figure 2-13). Studies of the comparative prognostic value of LVEF indicate that it is superior to other variables, including the history, physical examination, ECG, and cardiac serum enzyme data, as well as clinical prognostic indices. Because it is so powerful a predictor of prognosis, it is recommended that LVEF be measured in all MI patients before hospital discharge.

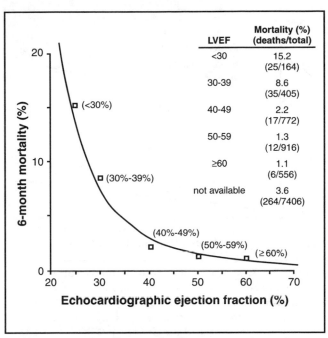

LVEF	Mortality (%) (deaths/total)
<30	15.2 (25/164)
30-39	8.6 (35/405)
40-49	2.2 (17/772)
50-59	1.3 (12/916)
≥60	1.1 (6/556)
not available	3.6 (264/7406)

Figure 2-13: Plot of 6-month all-cause mortality in five categories of echocardiographic left ventricular ejection fraction (LVEF). The ejection fraction-mortality curve exhibits a hyperbolic trend with an upturn in mortality occurring at values of less than 40%. With permission from Volpi et al, *Circulation* 1993;88:416-429.

Exercise Testing and Stress Imaging

The safety and utility of early post-MI treadmill exercise testing for risk stratification was established more than 20 years ago. The standard test employs a submaximal stress (treadmill or bicycle) based on variable end points, including 70% to 80% of age-predicted maximum heart rate, 5 to 6 METs (multiples of resting oxygen consumption), or absolute heart rate less than 130 beats/

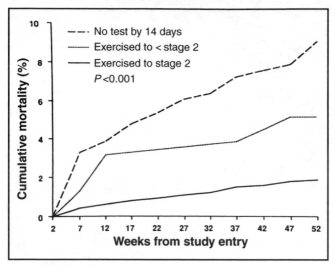

Figure 2-14: Mortality of patients in conservative strategy who did not perform exercise test compared with the mortality of those who were able to complete only one or both stages of low-level predischarge exercise test (*P* <0.001). With permission from Chaitman et al, *Am J Cardiol* 1993;71:131-138.

minute. In addition to identification of high-risk patients by ischemic ST-segment depression, factors associated with poor prognosis during submaximal testing include inability to perform or complete the test, impaired blood pressure response, ventricular tachycardia, and angina. As indicated in Figure 2-14 from the TIMI II thrombolysis trial, mortality at 52 weeks was lowest in post-MI patients able to complete a low-level exercise test and highest in those unable to perform the test. All patients in this study received thrombolytic therapy, and the gradations between posthospital mortality and exercise test results are similar to those found in reports from the prethrombolytic era. Exercise testing can also assess the adequacy of therapy, provide a basis for postdischarge

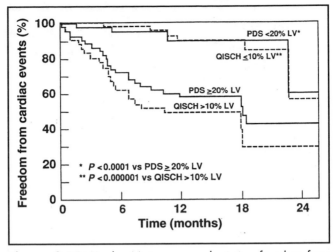

Figure 2-15: Kaplan-Meier curves depicting freedom from cardiac events based on the total left ventricular (LV) perfusion defect size (PDS) and the quantified extent of LV ischemia (QISCH). With permission from Mahmarian, *Cardiol Clin* 1995;13:355-378.

activity recommendations, and impart reassurance to the patient. With shortened hospital stay after uncomplicated MI, predischarge testing may be performed as early as day 3.

Although it has been reported that early symptom-limited testing can identify more patients at risk for future cardiac events than low-level testing, the most widely used method with the greatest record of safety and accuracy is the submaximal form.

Because post-MI outcomes are related to residual ischemia and LVEF, stress imaging studies, which can measure both variables, have excellent predictive results, which exceed the results of exercise testing and even coronary angiography for posthospital clinical course. Figure 2-15 depicts the frequency of recurrent cardiac

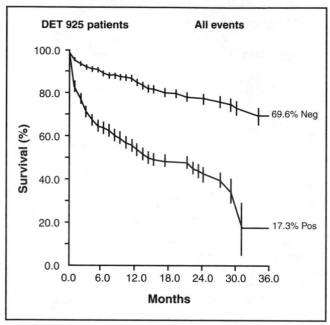

Figure 2-16: Cumulative event-free survival rates (including all events: death, reinfarction, angina, bypass, and angioplasty) in patients with negative (Neg) and positive (Pos) dipyridamole echocardiography test (DET) results. With permission from Picano et al, *Am J Med* 1993;95:608-618.

events in post-MI patients in relation to total perfusion defect size (by total thallium perfusion defect) and extent of residual ischemia (by reversible thallium perfusion defect). In this study, multivariate analysis revealed that LVEF and residual ischemia were the best predictors of hard events (death, recurrent MI) and total events (death, MI, unstable angina, heart failure) and improved risk stratification over that of clinical and angiographic data. Echocardiography provides similar quantitation of cardiac variables and risk stratification. In a study of more

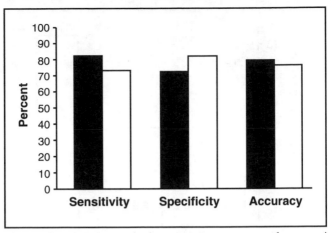

Figure 2-17: Bar graph showing sensitivity, specificity, and accuracy of contractile reserve (solid bars) and biphasic response (open bars) during exercise echocardiography for predicting functional recovery. With permission from Lancellotti et al, *J Am Coll Cardiol* 2003;41:1142-1147.

than 900 post-MI patients evaluated by dipyridamole (Persantine®) echocardiography, a new left ventricular wall motion abnormality indicative of ischemia was the most powerful predictor of subsequent events (Figure 2-16). In the early post-MI setting, pharmacologic echocardiography has generally been preferred over exercise or dobutamine (Dobutrex®) stress for risk stratification because of its safety and accuracy without undue stress. However, the latter methods have also been found safe and useful.

The use of echocardiography to predict functional recovery of regional myocardium in post-MI patients undergoing revascularization was recently extended by analysis of wall motion during exercise (Figure 2-17). Contractile reserve and a biphasic response (initial improvement of segmental wall motion and subsequent deteriora-

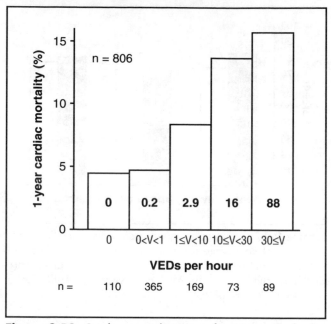

Figure 2-18: Cardiac mortality rate in five categories for frequency of ventricular ectopic depolarizations (VEDs) determined by 24-hour Holter recording before discharge (n denotes the number of patients in the total population and in each category). Of 819 patients with Holter recordings, 13 were lost to follow-up during the first year after hospitalization. The numbers within each of the boxes denote the median frequency of ventricular ectopy. With permission from *N Engl J Med* 1983;309:331-336.

tion) of ischemic myocardium during supine exercise echocardiography were the best predictors of recovery of contractile function in this study of 114 patients. This is the first report of the utility of a biphasic response during exercise echocardiography, a finding previously limited to observation during dobutamine echocardiography.

Noninvasive test selection for risk stratification is based on a number of factors. All available methods are potentially useful for this purpose. The greater predictive accuracy of imaging modalities is accompanied by increased complexity and cost. Submaximal treadmill exercise testing provides sufficient data for management of most patients, while a stress-imaging method is indicated in selected patients. These include patients who cannot exercise, patients with baseline ECG abnormalities that preclude interpretation of the exercise ECG, and patients with moderate or severely depressed LVEF in whom detection of residual ischemia will alter management.

Ventricular Arrhythmias

Ventricular arrhythmias in the peri-MI period, after the first 48 hours, represent persistent electrical instability and are predictors of postdischarge mortality. The frequency and complexity (multifocal, runs) of ventricular ectopic beats, detected predischarge by telemetry, ambulatory monitoring, or exercise testing, correlate with late sudden death and total mortality. In their study of 866 patients who had 24-hour ambulatory monitoring before discharge, the Multicenter Postinfarction Research Group demonstrated that 1-year mortality increased as the frequency of ventricular ectopy rose (Figure 2-18). However, while these arrhythmias had independent predictive value, their significance was markedly amplified in the presence of left ventricular dysfunction. Further, impaired LVEF (<40%) was a more important predictor of mortality than frequent ventricular ectopy ($\geq$10 depolarizations/hr), with a relative risk of 2.4 for the former compared with 1.6 for the latter.

The interaction of ventricular arrhythmias and left ventricular dysfunction was also shown in the Multicenter Investigation of the Limitation of Infarct Size (MILIS) study of 533 post-MI patients. Ventricular ectopic activity of >10 beats/hr was identified as the most important arrhythmic predictor of late sudden death, and LVEF

Table 2-7: Risk of Sudden Death After Myocardial Infarction

Group	Sudden Death (Follow-up 18 ± 8 mo)
LVEF ≥0.40	2%
LVEF <0.40	10%
≥10 VPB/hr, LVEF ≥0.40	8%
≥10 VPB/hr, LVEF <0.40	18%

LVEF = left ventricular ejection fraction,
VPB = ventricular premature beats
Adapted with permission from Mukharji et al, *Am J Cardiol* 1984;54:31-36.

<40% was the next strongest predictor. Table 2-7 shows the rates of sudden death at 18 months in relation to the presence or absence of these factors. Absence of both factors was associated with a low adverse outcome, which rose equally with the presence of either predictor, while the combination conferred a ninefold increase in risk of sudden death. Management of patients with asymptomatic, high-grade ventricular ectopy following MI is presented in Chapter 3.

Recent Prognostic Models

Although they provided important models of risk stratification, the applicability of early studies is limited by the major advances in contemporary management of patients with acute MI. In order to provide a contemporary approach, predictive scores have been developed from recent, large clinical trials of patients with ACS, and they have confirmed the validity of prognostication from clinically accessible variables in the modern era.

GUSTO-I

In the GUSTO-I thrombolytic trial of more than 40,000 patients, the prognostic importance of 16 demographic and clinical characteristics was determined by multivariate analysis. A striking finding of this study, as shown in Figure 2-19, is that five variables (age, systolic blood pressure, Killip class, heart rate, and MI location) accounted for more than 90% of the 30-day mortality in this group. The effect of age on both short-term and long-term post-MI risk has become increasingly important as the growing elderly population contributes a greater proportion of patients to the total MI population. In this regard, it has recently been reported that the recommended tests for post-MI risk stratification are significantly less likely to be performed in the elderly than in younger patients, as is demonstrated by Figures 2-20 and 2-21 from the Medicare database of more than 190,000 patients.

TIMI Risk Score for NSTEMI

Based on data from more than 5,000 patients in several major trials, the TIMI risk score for unstable angina/NSTEMI was derived by multivariate logistic regression analysis of multiple clinical variables. This method yielded seven simple risk factors that could be applied dichotomously to produce a score that predicted the 14-day probability of death and ischemic events. The predictor variables were: age ≥65 years, ≥3 coronary artery disease risk factors, prior coronary artery disease (≥50% stenosis), ST-segment deviation on presentation, ≥2 anginal events in the previous 24 hours, aspirin use in the previous 7 days, and elevated serum cardiac markers. The total number of events comprising the end points (all-cause mortality, new or recurrent MI, or urgent revascularization) rose significantly with increasing score (Figure 2-22). In this analysis, it was also shown that the rate of increase in events was lower in patients treated with enoxaparin (Lovenox®) than in patients treated with unfractionated heparin

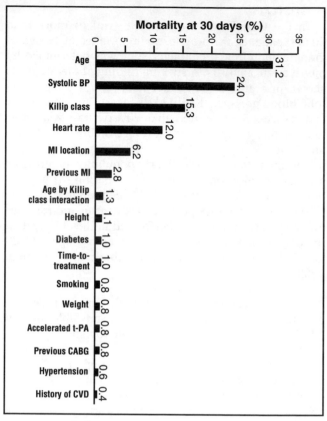

Figure 2-19: A multivariate mode of mortality at 30 days in the Global Use of Strategies to Open Occluded Arteries in Acute Coronary Syndromes (GUSTO-I) trial. The listed factors provide the relative importance in affecting mortality among the 41,021 patients studied. Adapted from Topol EJ, Van de Werf FJ: Chapter 17. Acute myocardial infarction. Early diagnosis and management. In: Topol E, ed: *Textbook of Cardiovascular Medicine*. Philadelphia, Lippincott-Raven, 1998:395-435, and data adapted from Lee et al, *Circulation* 1995; 91:1659-1668.

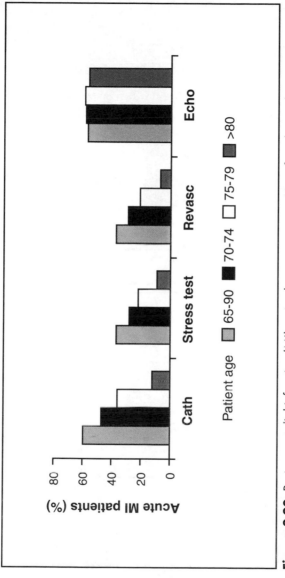

Figure 2-20: Post-myocardial infarction (MI) testing by age category. Use of cardiac catheterization, stress testing, revascularization, and echocardiography within 60 days of MI. With permission from Alexander et al, *Am Heart J* 2001;142:37-42.

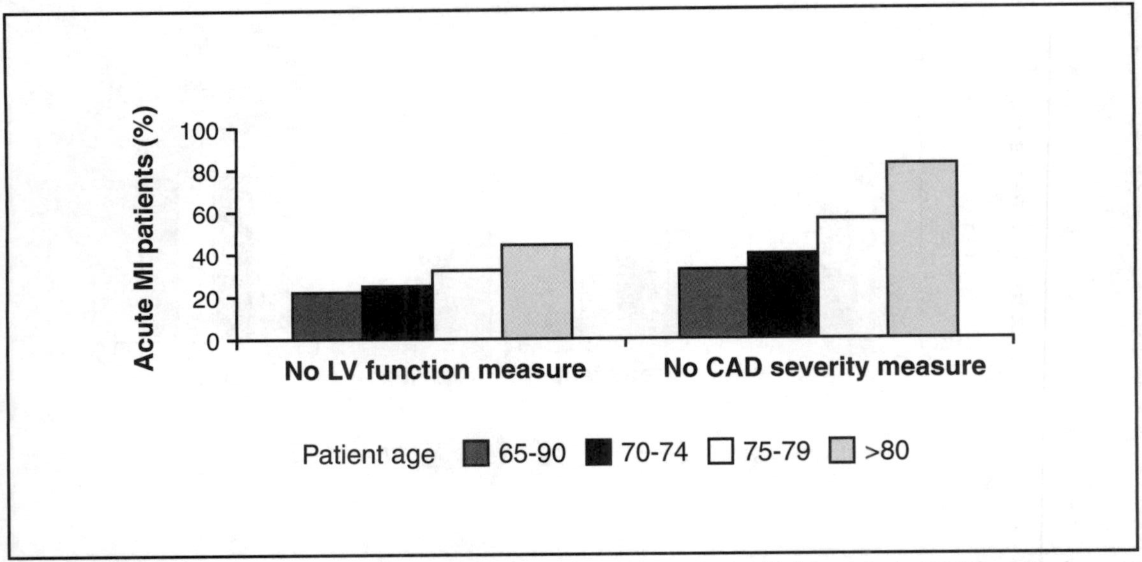

Figure 2-21: Assessment of coronary artery disease (CAD) severity and left ventricular (LV) function by age category. The proportion of patients who undergo no assessment of LV function or CAD severity is shown by age category. With permission from Alexander et al, *Am Heart J* 2001;142:37-42.

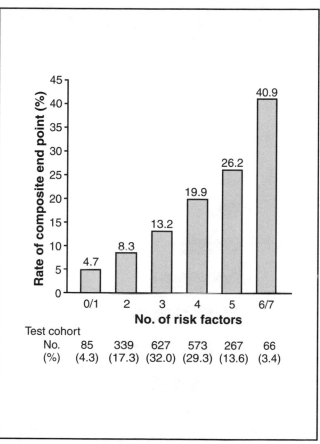

Figure 2-22: Thrombolysis in Myocardial Infarction (TIMI) risk score. Rates of all-cause mortality, myocardial infarction, and severe recurrent ischemia prompting urgent revascularization through 14 days after randomization were calculated for various patient subgroups based on the number of risk factors present in the test cohort (the unfractionated heparin group in the TIMI IIB trial; n =1957). Event rates increased significantly as the TIMI risk score increased (*P* <0.001 x 2 for trend). With permission from Antman et al, *JAMA* 2000;284:835-842.

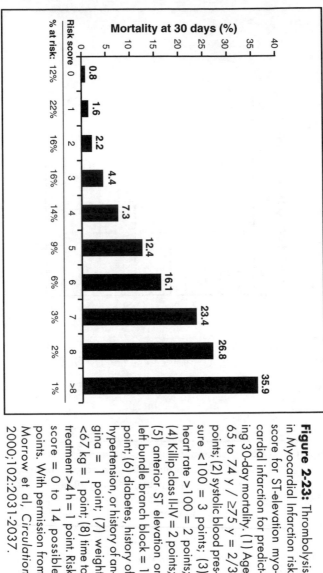

Figure 2-23: Thrombolysis in Myocardial Infarction risk score for ST-elevation myocardial infarction for predicting 30-day mortality. (1) Age 65 to 74 y / ≥75 y = 2/3 points; (2) systolic blood pressure <100 = 3 points; (3) heart rate >100 = 2 points; (4) Killip class II-IV = 2 points; (5) anterior ST elevation or left bundle branch block = 1 point; (6) diabetes, history of hypertension, or history of angina = 1 point; (7) weight <67 kg = 1 point; (8) time to treatment >4 h = 1 point. Risk score = 0 to 14 possible points. With permission from Morrow et al, *Circulation* 2000;102:2031-2037.

(Calciparine®, Liquaemin®), indicating that the TIMI risk score could be used in therapeutic decision making.

TIMI Risk Score for STEMI

The TIMI risk score for patients with STEMI is based on analysis of data from the Intravenous nPA for Treatment of Infarcting Myocardium Early-2 (InTIME 2) trial of more than 14,000 patients eligible for thrombolysis. Using logistic regression analysis of multiple clinical variables, this score was developed in a manner similar to that for the NSTEMI score. The STEMI score,which was obtained from the arithmetic sum of eight baseline factors (Figure 2-23), accounted for 97% of the power of this model to predict 30-day mortality. Within the overall mortality of 6.7%, a graded difference up to 40-fold was identified by the TIMI score. Mortality was <1% with a score of 0, while a score >8 predicted >35% mortality. The utility of the score was sustained over a 1-year interval.

The Open Artery Hypothesis

The 'open artery hypothesis' refers to the concept that late restoration of patency of the infarct-related coronary artery (IRA) reduces long-term mortality and morbidity after acute MI. It has been advanced as a rationale for direct coronary angiography in all post-MI patients to ensure restoration of flow in the IRA by coronary intervention when appropriate. Proposed mechanisms of benefit include limitation of left ventricular remodeling, maintenance of electrical stability, and supply of collateral blood flow. Although improved outcomes are supported by some observational studies (Table 2-8), there are no controlled trial data on this issue. The largest retrospective analysis of this question (GUSTO-I) revealed that IRA patency was not independently associated with reduced mortality at 1 year (Table 2-8). Resolution of this question awaits the results of the Occluded Artery Trial (OAT), a prospective, randomized trial that is testing the hypothesis that opening the IRA within 3 to 28 days after acute

**Table 2-8: Relationship Between Status of
the Infarct-related Artery
and Long-term Mortality**

Author	Year	No.	Initial therapy
Cigarroa et al	1989	179	Mixed
Gohlke et al	1991	102	NA
Galvani et al	1993	172	Mixed
White et al	1994	305	Thrombolytics
Lamas et al	1995	946	Mixed
Welty et al	1996	479	Mixed
Brodie et al	1996	565	Primary percutaneous transluminal coronary angioplasty
Puma et al*	1999	11,228	Thrombolytics

* Data reflect unadjusted mortality rates. After adjustment for baseline clinical factors and left ventricular ejection fraction, open IRA was not independently associated with improved 1-year survival.

MI in asymptomatic patients with LVEF ≤50% reduces mortality and morbidity over a 3-year follow-up interval.

Summary

The goals of management for survivors of acute MI are to prevent mortality and morbidity and to restore each patient to optimal functional status. All patients should receive

Follow-up (mo)	Mortality (%)		Relative risk reduction (%)
	Patent IRA	Occluded IRA	
47	0	18	100
51	13	17	24
43	1	17	94
39	4.5	9.5	53
42	11	24	54
34	4	17	76
64	7.7	15	49
12	3.3	8.8*	65

Mixed = initial therapy included thrombolytic therapy and no thrombolysis, NA = not available, IRA = infarct-related artery

With permission from Sadanandan et al, *Am Heart J* 2001;142:411-421.

comprehensive secondary prevention by modification of atherosclerotic risk factors and cardioprotective drug therapy (Chapters 3 through 6). Selected patients with high prognostic risk may also benefit from myocardial revascularization. The studies cited in this chapter demonstrate that high-risk patients can be reliably identified by a variety of methods that combine clinical assessment with noninvasive

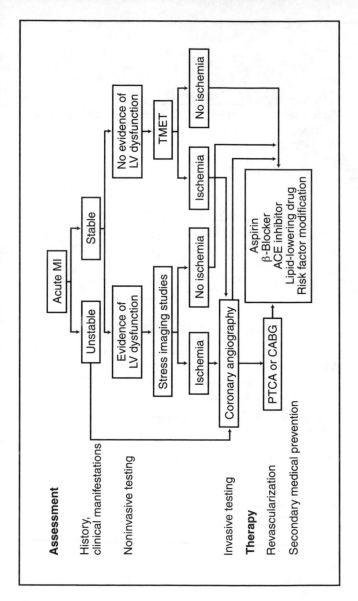

Figure 2-24: Algorithm for predischarge management of patients who have had an acute myocardial infarction (MI). Management of asymptomatic patients should generally follow the simple strategy outlined. This approach entails risk stratification and initiation of preventive therapy in all patients before discharge. It proceeds systematically from assessment by clinical status and left ventricular (LV) function, which determines the noninvasive method for detection of myocardial ischemia. The results of the latter, in turn, provide the basis for selection of medical therapy only or additional evaluation by invasive study (coronary angiography) and possible myocardial revascularization. Patients with persistent or recurrent symptoms of cardiac failure, ischemia, or ventricular arrhythmias (unstable condition) should undergo direct coronary angiography. If anatomy is suitable for revascularization, they are candidates for myocardial revascularization (percutaneous transluminal coronary angioplasty [PTCA] or coronary artery bypass graft surgery [CABG]). There are two subgroups of patients without evidence of LV dysfunction. The first subgroup would include those patients who appear stable clinically after an acute MI. These patients should undergo submaximal treadmill testing. The second subgroup consists of patients in whom there is evidence of LV dysfunction (shown by previous history, initial clinical manifestations, or presence of extensive anterior MI). In this second subgroup, assessment of LV function should be made by echocardiography. If the LV function is adequate (ejection fraction ≥40%), treadmill exercise testing (TMET) should be performed to detect myocardial ischemia. If the ejection fraction is less than 40%, a stress imaging study should be obtained to apply the most sensitive means of detecting ischemia in this high-risk group. Further management should be based on the presence or absence of ischemia. If no ischemia is present, patients should receive preventive therapy, consisting of coronary risk factor modification, aspirin, and individual factors; patients should undergo coronary angiography, and those with suitable anatomy are candidates for revascularization. They should also receive the same nonpharmacologic and pharmacologic therapy as that given to patients with no ischemia for prevention of recurrent coronary events. With permission from Deedwania et al, *Arch Intern Med* 1997;157:273-280.

testing to determine which patients are candidates for coronary angiography. Simple clinical variables are immediately accessible as early predictors of short-term and long-term risk. The two critical components of noninvasive risk stratification are the assessment of residual left ventricular function, which is usually performed by echocardiography, and the identification of jeopardized myocardium, which is attained from evidence of ischemia on treadmill testing or cardiac stress imaging. Indications for the latter studies are noted earlier in this chapter. This progressive approach affords the most rational, accurate, and cost-effective strategy for the selection of patients for coronary angiography. One such algorithm is presented in Figure 2-24. It is emphasized that, in this, as in all aspects of patient care, such algorithms serve as a guideline, and final management decisions require the physician's judgment based on the individual factors in each patient.

References

Ahumada GG: Identification of patients who do not require beta antagonists after myocardial infarction. *Am J Med* 1984;76:900-904.

Alexander KP, Galanos AN, Jollis JG, et al: Post-myocardial infarction risk stratification in elderly patients. *Am Heart J* 2001;142:37-42.

Antman EM, Cohen M, Bernink PJ, et al: The TIMI risk score for unstable angina/non-ST elevation MI: a method for prognostication and therapeutic decision making. *JAMA* 2000;284:835-842.

Antman EM, Tanasijevic MJ, Thompson B, et al: Cardiac-specific troponin I levels to predict the risk of mortality in patients with acute coronary syndromes. *N Engl J Med* 1996;335:1342-1349.

Braunwald E, Antman EM, Beasley JW, et al: ACC/AHA 2002 guideline update for the management of patients with unstable angina and non-ST-segment elevation myocardial infarction: a report of the American College of Cardiology/American Heart Association Task Force on Practice Guidelines (Committee on the Management of Patients With Unstable Angina). *J Am Coll Cardiol* 2002;40:1366-1374. Available at: http://www.acc.org/clinical/guidelines/unstable/unstable.pdf. Accessed on May 16, 2003.

Cannon C, Braunwald E: Chapter 10. Unstable angina. In: Braunwald E, Zipes D, Libby P, eds: *Heart Disease*. 6th ed. Philadelphia, WB Saunders, 2001.

Cannon CP, McCabe CH, Stone PH, et al: The electrocardiogram predicts one-year outcome of patients with unstable angina and non-Q wave myocardial infarction: results of the TIMI III Registry ECG Ancillary Study. Thrombolysis in Myocardial Ischemia. *J Am Coll Cardiol* 1997;30:133-140.

Cannon CP, Weintraub WS, Demopoulos LA, et al: Comparison of early invasive and conservative strategies in patients with unstable coronary syndromes treated with the glycoprotein IIb/IIIa inhibitor tirofiban. *N Engl J Med* 2001;344:1879-1887.

Chaitman BR, McMahon RP, Terrin M, et al: Impact of treatment strategy on predischarge exercise test in the Thrombolysis in Myocardial Infarction (TIMI) II Trial. *Am J Cardiol* 1993;71:131-138.

Deedwania PC, Amsterdam EA, Vagelos RH: Evidence-based, cost-effective risk stratification and management after myocardial infarction. California Cardiology Working Group on Post-MI Management. *Arch Intern Med* 1997;157:273-280.

Forrester JS, Diamond GA, Swan HJ: Correlative classification of clinical and hemodynamic function after acute myocardial infarction. *Am J Cardiol* 1977;39:137-145.

Francis GS, Alpert JS, eds: *Coronary Care*. 2nd ed. Philadelphia, Lippincott Williams & Wilkins, 1995:663-668.

Henning H: Chapter 38. Prognosis of acute myocardial infarction. In: Francis GS, Alpert JS, eds: *Coronary Care*. 2nd ed. Philadelphia, Lippincott Williams & Wilkins, 1995:689-740.

Kao W, Khaja F, Goldstein S, et al: Cardiac event rate after non-Q-wave acute myocardial infarction and the significance of its anterior location. *Am J Cardiol* 1989;64:1236-1242.

Killip T 3rd, Kimball JT: Treatment of myocardial infarction in a coronary care unit. A two year experience with 250 patients. *Am J Cardiol* 1967;20:457-464.

Lancellotti P, Hoffer EP, Pierard LA: Detection and clinical usefulness of a biphasic response during exercise echocardiography early after myocardial infarction. *J Am Coll Cardiol* 2003;41:1142-1147.

Lee KL, Woodlief LH, Topol EJ, et al: Predictors of 30-day mortality in the era of reperfusion for acute myocardial infarction.

Results from an international trial of 41,021 patients. GUSTO-I Investigators. *Circulation* 1995;91:1659-1668.

Mahmarian JJ: Prediction of myocardium at risk. Clinical significance during acute infarction and in evaluating subsequent prognosis. *Cardiol Clin* 1995;13:355-378.

Morrow DA, Antman EM, Charlesworth A, et al: TIMI risk score for ST-elevation myocardial infarction: A convenient, bedside, clinical score for risk assessment at presentation: An Intravenous nPA for Treatment of Infarcting Myocardium Early II trial substudy. *Circulation* 2000;102:2031-2037.

Morrow DA, Rifai N, Antman EM, et al: C-reactive protein is a potent predictor of mortality independently of and in combination with troponin T in acute coronary syndromes: a TIMI 11A substudy. Thrombolysis in Myocardial Infarction. *J Am Coll Cardiol* 1998;31:1460-1465.

Mukharji J, Rude RE, Poole WK, et al: Risk factors for sudden death after acute myocardial infarction: two-year follow-up. *Am J Cardiol* 1984;54:31-36.

Norris RM, Caughey DE, Deeming LW, et al: Coronary prognostic index for predicting survival after recovery from acute myocardial infarction. *Lancet* 1970;2:485-487.

Nyman I, Areskog M, Areskog NH, et al: Very early risk stratification by electrocardiogram at rest in men with suspected unstable coronary heart disease. The RISC Study Group. *J Intern Med* 1993;234:293-301.

Peel AA, Semple T, Wang I, et al: A coronary prognostic index for grading severity of infarction. *Br Heart J* 1962;24:745-760.

Picano E, Landi P, Bolognese L, et al: Prognostic value of dipyridamole echocardiography early after uncomplicated myocardial infarction: a large-scale, multicenter trial. The EPIC Study Group. *Am J Med* 1993;95:608-618.

Risk stratification and survival after myocardial infarction. *N Engl J Med* 1983;309:331-336.

Ryan TJ, Antman EM, Brooks NH, et al: ACC/AHA guidelines for the management of patients with acute myocardial infarction: 1999 update: a report of the American College of Cardiology/ American Heart Association Task Force on Practice Guidelines (Committee on Management of Acute Myocardial Infarction). Available at: http://www.acc.org. Accessed on May 16, 2003.

Sadanandan S, Buller C, Menon V, et al: The late open artery hypothesis—a decade later. *Am Heart J* 2001;142:411-421.

Topol EJ, Van de Werf FJ: Chapter 17. Acute myocardial infarction. Early diagnosis and management. In: Topol E, ed: *Textbook of Cardiovascular Medicine.* Philadelphia, Lippincott-Raven, 1998:395-435.

Topol EJ, ed: *Textbook of Cardiovascular Medicine.* Philadelphia, Lippincott-Raven Publishers, 1997:341-364.

Volpi A, De Vita C, Franzosi MG, et al: Determinants of 6-month mortality in survivors of myocardial infarction after thrombolysis. Results of the GISSI-2 data base. The Ad hoc Working Group of the Gruppo Italiano per lo Studio della Sopravvivenza nell'Infarto Miocardico (GISSI)-2 Data Base. *Circulation* 1993; 88:416-429.

Chapter 3

Cardioprotective Drug Therapy

S everal pharmacologic agents are now established as standard treatment for secondary prevention of recurrent coronary heart disease (CHD) events in patients who have had an acute myocardial infarction (MI). Because of their demonstrated efficacy in decreasing long-term CHD morbidity and mortality in randomized clinical trials, these drugs are referred to as 'cardioprotective.' Moreover, they exert their beneficial effects on secondary prevention irrespective of conventional symptomatic indications for their use. They include aspirin, angiotensin-converting enzyme (ACE) inhibitors, and β-blockers and are the major subjects of this chapter. Consideration will also be given to calcium-channel blockers (CCBs), nitrates, the current status of hormone replacement therapy (HRT), and the role of long-term antiarrhythmic modalities. Lipid-lowering drugs are considered in Chapter 4.

Trends in Therapy After Myocardial Infarction

An area of continuing concern in the management of post-MI patients is the inadequate use of proven cardioprotective drug therapy, a phenomenon that has been referred to as the 'knowledge-practice gap.' This problem has been consistently documented in large-scale studies, and, although there has been recent improvement, significant opportunity remains for further gains. A National Registry of Myocardial Infarction report on annual trends in discharge medications for patients after acute MI between 1994 and 1999 revealed that aspirin was the most frequently used drug, increasing slightly from 75% of patients in 1994 to 80% in 1999. The administration of β-blockers, on the other hand, increased considerably, from just over 40% of patients to 65%. Although the use of ACE inhibitors remained low, there was a gradual rise from 25% to almost 40%. On the other hand, post-MI use of CCBs has decreased from more than 30% to less than 20%. Application of antiarrhythmic drugs remained minimal at 5%.

Aspirin and Other Antiplatelet Agents

Aspirin

The rupture of an atherosclerotic plaque is the initiating process in acute MI. Circulating platelets are exposed to thrombogenic factors within the plaque, leading to platelet activation, adhesion, aggregation, and the formation of a flow-limiting thrombus. The efficacy of aspirin as an antiplatelet agent is primarily related to its interference with the biosynthesis of the cyclic prostanoid, thromboxane A_2, a potent platelet activator and vasospastic mediator. Aspirin is the first medication given to patients on presentation to the emergency department for suspected acute coronary syndromes (ACS). The drug is rapidly absorbed from the stomach and reaches appreciable plasma levels in 20 minutes. Platelet inhibition develops in approximately 1 hour. Because of the development of thrombosis as a final pathway for coronary occlusion and resultant MI, it is rational to administer aspirin as early as possible and to continue its use indefinitely. Pharmacodynamic studies indicate that medium-dose aspirin (162 mg, one half of an adult aspirin) inhibits thromboxane A_2 synthesis and diminishes platelet activity.

Despite ample demonstration of aspirin's efficacy in secondary prevention, a survey found that its use in patients with CHD increased from 5% to only 26% from 1980 to 1996. Cardiologists reported aspirin use of only 37% in patients with CHD, and this practice was even lower for internists (20%), family physicians (18%), and general practitioners (11%) from 1993 to 1996. Several trials have demonstrated the efficacy of aspirin in modifying short-term and long-term mortality in MI. In the Second International Study of Infarct Survival (ISIS-2), for example, when compared with placebo, 160 mg of aspirin within 24 hours of acute MI reduced mortality by 23%, nonfatal reinfarction by 49%, and nonfatal stroke by 46% (Figure 3-1). This trial established the benefit of aspirin in acute MI. It has also been demonstrated that aspirin is incrementally beneficial when given in conjunction with thrombolytic agents. Other studies of aspirin initiated early or late after acute MI indicate a 5% to 40% reduction in cardiac mortality and a 10% to 60% reduction in nonfatal infarction. Nonfatal stroke rate has also been reduced by approximately 40%. A meta-analysis by the Antiplatelet Trialists, comprising 100,000 patients in whom aspirin was used for long-term treatment after acute MI and other high-risk cardiovascular conditions, demonstrated a decrease in vascular death of approximately 16% and a decrease in nonfatal MI or stroke of 33%. These results occurred without regard to age, gender, or presence of hypertension or diabetes.

Warfarin

Several long-term anticoagulant studies have demonstrated efficacy of oral anticoagulants following acute MI. For example, in the Warfarin Reinfarction Study (WARIS), warfarin (Coumadin®) decreased mortality by 24% compared with placebo over several years, with decreases of 34% in reinfarction and more than 50% in stroke. Several studies directly comparing aspirin with anticoagulants for long-term postinfarction prophylaxis

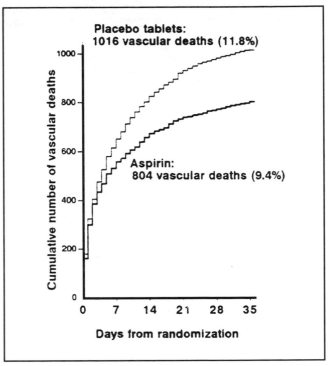

Figure 3-1: International Study of Infarct Survival (ISIS) results showing all patients allocated active aspirin vs all allocated placebo tablets. Adapted from *Lancet* 1988;2:349-360, with permission.

showed equivalency, although there was a higher frequency of bleeding with the anticoagulants and more frequent gastrointestinal side effects with aspirin.

Clopidogrel and Ticlopidine

Clopidogrel (Plavix®) and ticlopidine (Ticlid®) are thienopyridine derivatives that inhibit platelet aggregation by a mechanism different from that of aspirin. These drugs block the platelet adenosine diphosphate receptor,

81

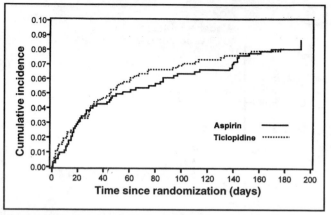

Figure 3-2: Results of the Study of Ticlopidine versus Aspirin After Myocardial Infarction (STAMI) showing lack of difference in cumulative incidence curve for primary end points, aspirin vs ticlopidine. From Scrutinio et al, *J Am Coll Cardiol* 2001; 37:1259-1265, with permission.

which amplifies platelet activation. Clopidogrel does not have the leukopenic side effect of ticlopidine.

Studies of aspirin, ticlopidine, or clopidogrel after acute MI have been frequently coupled with thrombolytic therapy. In one study of ticlopidine vs aspirin after thrombolysis, 6-month follow-up revealed no difference between groups in the combined end points of death, recurrent infarction, stroke, and angina (Figure 3-2).

The Clopidogrel vs Aspirin in Patients at Risk for Ischemic Events trial (CAPRIE) compared aspirin (325 mg/d) with clopidogrel (75 mg/d) over an average of 2 years for prevention of combined events of vascular death, MI, or stroke in patients with a history of MI, stroke, or peripheral vascular disease. Event rates were slightly, but significantly, lower with clopidogrel (5.32% vs 5.83% per year, $P = 0.04$), but there was no significant difference in the subset of patients who had a prior MI. There were no

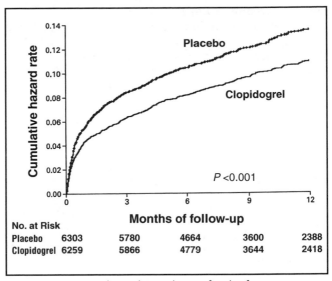

Figure 3-3: Cumulative hazard rates for the first primary outcome (death from cardiovascular causes, nonfatal myocardial infarction, or stroke) during the 12 months of the Clopidogrel in Unstable Angina to Prevent Recurrent Events (CURE) study. Both groups received aspirin. The results demonstrate the sustained effect of clopidogrel. From Yusuf et al, *N Engl J Med* 2001;345:494-502, with permission.

differences in adverse effects. Although there is no evidence that clopidogrel or ticlopidine is more effective than aspirin following ST-elevation MI, the recent Clopidogrel in Unstable Angina to Prevent Recurrent Events (CURE) (Figure 3-3) trial demonstrated superiority of clopidogrel plus aspirin compared with aspirin alone for long-term treatment of non-ST-elevation ACS. Patients on the two drugs had a 20% reduction (P <0.001) of the combined end point of death, recurrent ischemic events, rehospitalization, and revascularization during the 12-month follow-up period after the initial ACS.

Platelet Glycoprotein IIb/IIIa Blockers

The final pathway in platelet aggregation is mediated by the glycoprotein (GP) IIb/IIIa receptor, found exclusively on the surface of platelets and megakaryocytes. Through this receptor, fibrinogen combines with platelet aggregates to form the mature red thrombus, which is the culmination of the events initiated by plaque rupture. Platelet GPIIb/IIIa receptor inhibitors have been studied extensively in the treatment of acute MI, primarily as adjunctive agents with thrombolysis and coronary angioplasty/stenting in an effort to enhance and sustain reperfusion of the infarct-related artery. There has been limited evaluation of IIb/IIIa receptor inhibitors as isolated treatment after MI. These agents are usually administered for 48 to 72 hours during the acute coronary event. They are available only in intravenously administered forms and, therefore, cannot be used for long-term post-MI therapy.

Combinations of tirofiban (Aggrastat®) with aspirin vs heparin plus aspirin in the acute phase of unstable angina were shown to favor the IIb/IIIa-aspirin combination in 30-day mortality (2.3% vs 3.6%, $P = 0.02$). In the Platelet Receptor Inhibition in Ischemic Syndrome Management in Patients Limited by Unstable Signs and Symptoms (PRISM-PLUS) study of non-ST-elevation ACS, in which all patients received aspirin, tirofiban alone was associated with a higher 30-day mortality than heparin alone at 7 days. However, at 30 days and 6 months, with continued aspirin therapy in each case, early initiation of tirofiban plus heparin produced a better clinical outcome than either agent alone.

In longer studies, combination of a IIb/IIIa inhibitor with aspirin in ACS has produced equivocal results. In a 30-day follow-up study of more than 10,000 patients with non-ST-elevation ACS (Platelet Glycoprotein IIb/IIIa in Unstable Angina: Receptor Suppression Using Integrilin Therapy [PURSUIT] trial) eptifibatide (Integrilin®) administered for up to 72 hours reduced combined fatal and nonfatal MI. A recent meta-analysis of these and other trials of IIb/IIIa receptor antagonists in non-ST-elevation ACS demonstrated a significant decrease in 30-day mortality in patients with diabetes, especially in those undergoing percutaneous coronary interventions.

β-Blockers

β-Blockers have multiple properties that appear to have the potential to protect against recurrent myocardial ischemia and infarction. Their antiadrenergic effects lower blood pressure and heart rate, reduce shear stress due to decreased left ventricular (LV) dp/dt, decrease platelet aggregation, and lessen the permeability of the endothelium to atherogenic lipoproteins. Extensive clinical trials over the past 2 decades have demonstrated that β-blockade decreases post-MI mortality and, specifically, sudden cardiac death over several years (Figures 3-4, 3-5, 3-6, 3-7, and 3-8).

In the β-Blocker Heart Attack Trial (BHAT), 3,837 patients aged 30 to 69 years who had experienced at least one MI were followed up for 2 to 4 years after administration of propranolol (Inderal®) or placebo. The trial was stopped 9 months early. Over an average 24-month follow-up period, total mortality was 7.2% in the propranolol group and 9.8% in the placebo group. Sudden cardiac death was 3.3% in the propranolol group and 4.6% in the placebo group. Coronary incidence, defined as recurrent nonfatal reinfarction plus fatal CHD, was reduced by 23% in the propranolol group compared with placebo. Based on these results, the investigators concluded that in patients with no contraindications to β-blockers, treatment should be initiated and continued for at least 3 years.

Although BHAT demonstrated efficacy only for high-risk Q-wave MI patients compared with low-risk Q-wave MI patients and showed no significant effect in non-Q-wave MI patients (Figures 3-4 and 3-5), later studies have

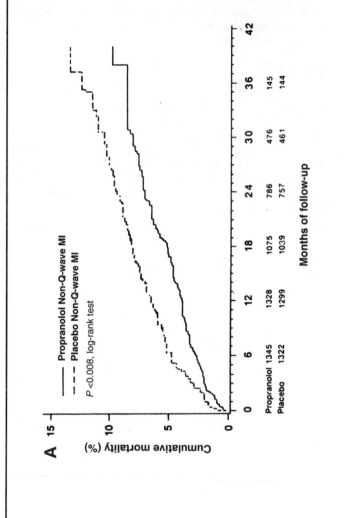

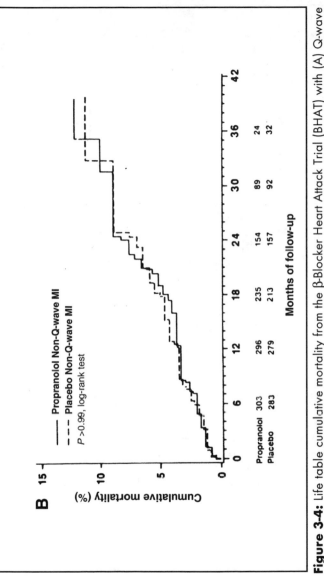

Figure 3-4: Life table cumulative mortality from the β-Blocker Heart Attack Trial (BHAT) with (A) Q-wave and (B) non-Q-wave myocardial infarction results. Only in the Q-wave group were β-blockers effective. From Gheorghiade et al, *Am J Cardiol* 1990;66:129-133, with permission.

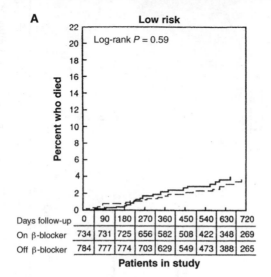

Days follow-up

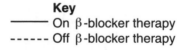

Key
——— On β-blocker therapy
- - - - - Off β-blocker therapy

Figure 3-5: Long-term mortality in the β-Blocker Heart Attack Trial (BHAT) for (A) low-risk, (B) medium-risk, and (C) high-risk patients: β-blocker vs placebo. Risk stratification was based on recurrent ischemic events, arrhythmias, congestive heart failure, or severe comorbidity during the first 12 months after acute myocardial infarction. Only in the high-risk group was there a favorable effect of β-blockers in this trial. From Viscoli et al, *Ann Intern Med* 1993;118:99-105, with permission.

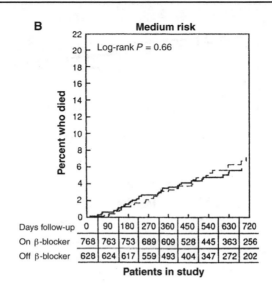

B   **Medium risk**

Log-rank *P* = 0.66

Days follow-up	0	90	180	270	360	450	540	630	720
On β-blocker	768	763	753	689	609	528	445	363	256
Off β-blocker	628	624	617	559	493	404	347	272	202

Patients in study

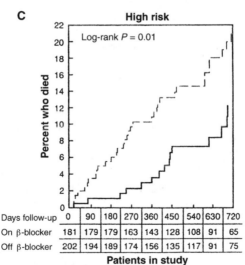

C   **High risk**

Log-rank *P* = 0.01

Days follow-up	0	90	180	270	360	450	540	630	720
On β-blocker	181	179	179	163	143	128	108	91	65
Off β-blocker	202	194	189	174	156	135	117	91	75

Patients in study

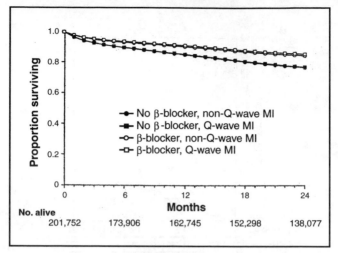

Figure 3-6: Adjusted probability of survival among patients with Q-wave and non-Q-wave myocardial infarction who received or did not receive β-blockers. The patients with Q-wave infarction and those with non-Q-wave infarction had similar benefit with β-blockade. From Gottlieb et al, *N Engl J Med* 1998;339:489-497, with permission.

shown a beneficial effect even in non-Q-wave MI patients (Figure 3-6). In this regard, a beneficial effect on sudden cardiac death is not evident with antiplatelet agents. The average reduction in total mortality with β-blockade is approximately 20%, or an absolute decrease from 10% to 8%, while sudden cardiac death is lowered by 32% to 50%.

The major studies demonstrating β-blocker efficacy after acute MI include trials of timolol (Blocadren®), propranolol, metoprolol (Lopressor®, Toprol XL®), and, most recently, carvedilol (Coreg®). They show that timolol decreased sudden cardiac death by almost 50%, metoprolol reduced mortality within 24 hours of symptoms by 40%, and propranolol decreased sudden cardiac death by 30%.

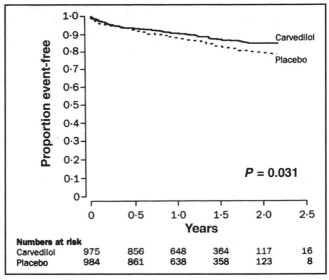

Figure 3-7: Outcomes in carvedilol- and placebo-treated patients in the Carvedilol Post Infarction Survival Control in Left Ventricular Dysfunction (CAPRICORN) trial. *Lancet* 2001;357: 1385-1390.

The Norwegian Timolol Trial involved 1,884 patients enrolled 7 to 28 days after MI and followed for a mean of 17 months. The cumulated death rate over 33 months was 7.7% in the timolol group and 13.9% in the placebo group, a reduction of 44%. The cumulated reinfarction rate was 14.4% in the timolol group and 20.1% in the placebo group. These results were highly significant, indicating that long-term treatment with timolol after acute MI reduced mortality and rates of reinfarction.

The Goteborg Metoprolol Trial evaluated 1,395 patients with suspected acute MI who were randomized to metoprolol or placebo at the time of hospital admission. Therapy was continued for a 90-day period, allowing evaluation of short-term benefits of β-blocker use. Dur-

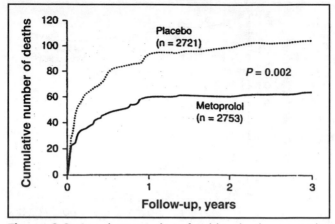

Figure 3-8: Cumulative number of sudden deaths reported in five postinfarction trials. From Kendall et al, *Ann Intern Med* 1995;123:358-367, with permission.

ing this period, mortality was 5.7% in the metoprolol group and 8.9% in the placebo group, a significant 36% decrease in the β-blocker group. Moreover, institution of metoprolol within 12 hours of admission beneficially influenced infarct development and infarct size during the first 3 days. Fewer episodes of ventricular fibrillation were seen in the metoprolol group (6 patients vs 17 patients in the placebo group). Among patients with mild-to-moderate congestive heart failure before randomization, 90-day mortality in the β-blocker group was 10% compared to 19% in the placebo group. At 1 year, the corresponding figures were 14% in the metoprolol group and 27% in the placebo group. All these results were significantly different, demonstrating the benefits of very early β-blocker intervention after an acute coronary event.

The Metoprolol in Acute Myocardial Infarction (MI-AMI) trial was an expanded trial (5,778 patients) based on the principles of the Goteborg trial. Metoprolol was administered within 24 hours of the development of symptoms suggesting acute MI, and therapy was continued for 15 days. The metoprolol-treated patients were matched with a placebo group. At the end of only 15 days, there was a 13% decrease in mortality in the metoprolol group (4.3% vs 4.9% in the placebo group), although the difference lacked significance. Among patients at higher risk, however, mortality reduction was significant (29%). In addition, the incidence of definite acute MI and peak serum enzyme activity was reduced in the β-blocker group. More patients were treated with antiarrhythmics in the placebo group, predominantly within the first 5 days.

The Lopressor Intervention Trial enrolled 2,395 patients after acute MI, with metoprolol intervention beginning 6 to 16 days after acute MI and follow-up lasting a year. This trial was terminated prematurely because of a progressive and marked decline in patient accession. After 1 year, there was no significant difference in deaths between the metoprolol and placebo groups (65 vs 62), but mortality in the placebo group was only 5.2%, roughly half that predicted at the outset. The results reflect the common finding in clinical trials that study power calculations based on anticipated mortality in a placebo group greatly overestimate mortality.

Carvedilol, a newer β-blocker with α-blocking properties, has demonstrated potent anti-ischemic, cardioprotective, and antioxidant properties. It has shown beneficial effects in LV dysfunction. A study of 151 patients with acute MI evaluated acute intravenous and long-term (6-month) oral treatment with carvedilol compared with placebo. The number of cardiac events in the carvedilol group was significantly lower than that in the placebo group (18 vs 31). Other improvements in the carvedilol group included greater stroke volume and diastolic filling of the left ventricle.

The recent Carvedilol Post Infarction Survival Control in Left Ventricular Dysfunction (CAPRICORN) trial evaluated 1,959 patients with a proven acute MI and LV ejection fraction (LVEF) <40%. Patients were randomized to carvedilol (to a maximum of 25 mg twice daily) or placebo. All patients were taking ACE inhibitors unless intolerant of these agents. Patients with clinical indications for β-blockers were excluded. Although there was no difference in the primary end point of all-cause mortality or hospital admission for cardiovascular problems after a mean of 1.3 years of follow-up, all-cause mortality alone was lower in the carvedilol group (12% vs 15%, $P = 0.03$ [Figure 3-7]). Cardiovascular mortality and nonfatal MI were also reduced in patients randomized to carvedilol.

Other end points that showed significant benefit of carvedilol in the CAPRICORN trial included decreases in sudden death (hazard ratio [HR] 0.74), cardiovascular-cause mortality (HR 0.75), nonfatal MI (HR 0.59), and all-cause mortality or nonfatal MI (HR 0.71). The reduction in deaths and recurrent MI was found during both acute and chronic phases of the study. These beneficial outcomes applied equally to patients with objective evidence of LV dysfunction.

In summary, the CAPRICORN trial differed from previous large-scale β-blocker trials because patient selection was based on decreased LVEF and the drug's sympathetic blocking profile was broader. The reduction in mortality and recurrent MI was within the range of previous β-blocker studies in MI patients. For example, in CAPRICORN, the number of patients who needed to be treated to prevent one death was 28. For the Goteborg, Norwegian Timolol, and BHAT trials, it was 32, 18, and 38, respectively.

CAPRICORN also differed from previous β-blocker trials in that the protocol mandated use of ACE inhibitors during the acute phase for at least 48 hours before carvedilol was initiated. This emphasizes the importance of using stable doses of ACE inhibitors as well as diuretics in congestive heart failure patients with acute MI before β-blockers are considered.

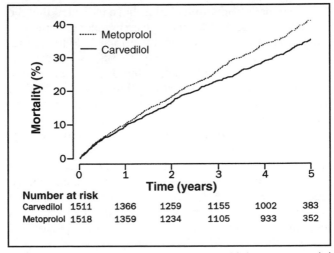

Figure 3-9: All-cause mortality in Carvedilol Or Metoprolol European Trial (COMET). From Poole-Wilson et al, *Lancet* 2003;362:7-13, with permission.

In the recently published Carvedilol Or Metoprolol European Trial (COMET) in patients with heart failure, carvedilol produced a significantly greater reduction in mortality than metoprolol tartrate. As shown in Figure 3-9, the benefit of carvedilol on mortality occurred early and continued to increase throughout the duration of the trial. COMET is the first head-to-head mortality trial comparing carvedilol, a nonselective β-blocking agent, with metoprolol, a cardioselective β-blocking agent. The multicenter, double-blind study included 3,029 patients with moderate to severe heart failure followed for a mean period of 58 months. The patients were on background therapy with an ACE inhibitor and a diuretic. Although COMET was not a specific post-MI trial, 41% of the patients had a history of MI, and more than 50% had ischemic heart disease.

Pooled data from clinical trials have indicated that the primary effect of β-blockers on decreased long-term mortality after acute MI has been due primarily to the reduction of sudden cardiac death (Figure 3-8). Some investigators have questioned whether the decrease in sudden cardiac death is a class effect of β-blockers or is limited to specific agents. For example, the four agents in the major studies described above are lipophilic. Hydrophilic agents such as atenolol (Tenormin®) and sotalol (Betapace®, Betapace AF™) have not shown long-term prophylactic properties in regard to sudden cardiac death.

Despite strong evidence that they provide cardioprotection after acute MI, β-blockers have been markedly underused in this country, with less than 50% of patients receiving these drugs, according to surveys performed as late as the mid-1990s. The recent incremental increase in β-blocker therapy in post-MI patients may be related partly to the active promotion of this class of drugs through practice guidelines. In addition, the Cardiac Arrhythmia Suppression Trial (CAST), which revealed the adverse effects of antiarrhythmic agents used for long-term prophylaxis after MI, increased attention to the benefits of β-blockers.

Part of the reluctance of physicians to use β-blockers is attributable to their *relative* contraindications, which include obstructive pulmonary disease, diabetes, and peripheral vascular disease. However, it is now recognized that patients in these groups are at high risk for coronary events, that many can tolerate β-blockers, and that they benefit from β-blockers as much as or more than other patients (Figures 3-10 and 3-11). Patients with compensated pulmonary disease should be given a trial of low-dose β-blocker therapy, which can be continued or increased according to tolerance. In patients with pulmonary disease and non-Q-wave MI, β-blocker therapy has reduced mortality significantly, based on recent clinical trial data. Patients with diabetes appear to have a more beneficial response in terms of decreased mortality compared with patients without diabetes. Clinical trials in post-MI patients with peripheral vascular disease have shown no increase in adverse effects on the latter condition in those on β-blocker therapy compared with placebo. In contrast to the former concern about the use of β-blockers in patients with LV dysfunction, these drugs are now a mainstay in the management of heart failure when used judiciously with other established therapy. Recent clinical trials in congestive heart failure from ischemic and nonischemic cardiomyopathy have shown that β-blockers provide additional benefits of improving survival and LV function. In summary, there are relatively few absolute contraindications to the use of β-blockers after acute MI. They include severe pulmonary dysfunction, severe congestive heart failure, and second-degree atrioventricular block or marked sinus bradycardia, in the absence of a cardiac pacemaker. Optimal dosing should reflect the doses administered in clinical trials showing efficacy.

A study by Phillips et al points out the health and economic benefits of increased β-blocker use after MI. A computer simulation of the US population was used to estimate the impact of increased use of these agents. Phillips et al calculated that initiating β-blocker use in all MI survivors without contraindications in the year 2000 and continuing therapy in these patients for 20 years would result in 4,300 fewer CHD deaths, 3,500 MIs prevented, and 45,000 life-years gained compared with current usage (as of 1999). If β-blockers were initiated in all suitable MI survivors in the years 2000 through 2020 with similar 20-year continuation, $18 million would be saved, and the result would be 72,000 fewer CHD deaths, 62,000 MIs prevented, and 447,000 life-years gained. Phillips et al calculated that restricting β-blockers to only 'ideal' use would reduce the economic impact of these agents by about 60%.

Angiotensin-converting Enzyme Inhibitors

Angiotensin II is a potent factor in the pathophysiology of atherosclerosis and coronary ischemic events. Acting

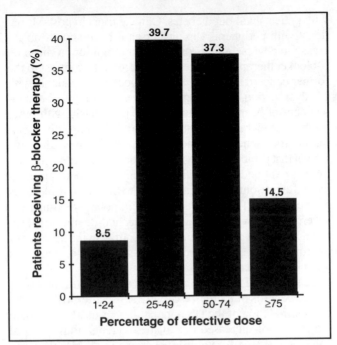

Figure 3-10: Distribution of infarct survivors with relative contra-indications to β-blockers who received β-blocker therapy (n = 362), according to the dose prescribed at hospital discharge. Dosages of β-blockers are shown as a percentage of effective dosage. From Barron et al, *Prev Cardiol* 1998;3:13-15, with permission.

through multiple pathways, this peptide exerts proinflammatory, prothrombotic, and atherogenic effects. The beneficial actions of ACE inhibitors are the result of inhibition of converting enzyme activity, reducing both production of angiotensin II and breakdown of bradykinin. These results provide ample protective mechanisms for ACE inhibitors, including decreased oxidative stress, improved fibrinolytic balance, reduced platelet activity, and lower plasminogen activator inhibitor levels. Angiotensin-converting enzyme in-

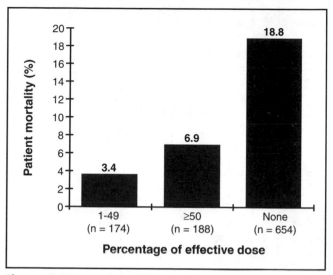

Figure 3-11: Unadjusted long-term mortality rates in patients with relative contraindications to β-blockers who survived the index hospitalization, according to the dose of β-blocker prescribed at hospital discharge. From Barron et al, *Prev Cardiol* 1998;3:13-15, with permission.

hibitors also decrease the migration of macrophages, reduce proliferation of vascular smooth muscle, reduce MI size, and retard detrimental LV remodeling. The beneficial effects of bradykinin include vasodilator actions and protective effects on vascular endothelium (Figure 3-12). The latter are mediated through an increase in nitric oxide (NO) production. In the past decade, the value of ACE inhibitors after acute MI has expanded from attenuation of LV remodeling to increased survival and decreased morbidity. Multitrial analysis of early use of ACE inhibitors in more than 100,000 patients (0 to 36 hours from onset of acute MI) demonstrates a reduction of 20% to 30% in mortality over 30 days, 80% of which was achieved in the first week of treatment.

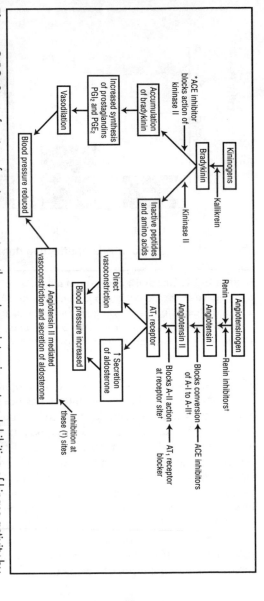

Figure 3-12: Sites of action of various agents on the renin-angiotensin system. Inhibition of kinase activity by angiotensin-converting enzyme (ACE) inhibition allows accumulation of vasodilator substances and contributes to blood pressure lowering. Angiotensin II (A-II) receptor blockade does not affect this system. A-I = angiotensin I, an inactive peptide; AT₁ = A-II receptor subtype I; PGE₂ = prostaglandin E₂; PGI₂ = prostacyclin. From Moser, J Am Coll Cardiol 1997;29:1414-1421, with permission.

100

The third Gruppo Italiano per lo Studio della Sopravvivenza nell'Infarto Miocardico (GISSI-3) trial evaluated the efficacy of treatment with lisinopril (Prinivil®, Zestril®), transdermal nitroglycerin, or their combination within 24 hours after acute MI in improving survival and ventricular function. Other therapies administered during the acute infarct period included thrombolysis (>70%), aspirin (>80%), and intravenous β-blockers (31%). A total of 19,394 patients was randomized; the dose of lisinopril was 5 mg initially and then 10 mg daily. The 6-week mortality was 6.3% in the ACE inhibitor group and 7.1% in the control group ($P = 0.03$), indicating a significant effect of ACE inhibitors, despite a high prevalence of complementary therapy (Figure 3-13). Echocardiography also revealed a smaller proportion of patients with LV ejection <35% in the lisinopril group. Additionally, in patients >70 years old and in women, lisinopril significantly reduced the combined end point of mortality and severe LV dysfunction. There was no excess of adverse effects related to study drugs.

The ISIS-4 trial also demonstrated a significant reduction in 5-week mortality after early initiation of an ACE inhibitor in acute MI. As in the GISSI-3 trial, 70% of patients also received thrombolytic therapy. Mortality reduction from ACE inhibitors was significant, but the absolute decrease was low (<1%). This trial revealed that evidence of higher risk, such as anterior MI, prior MI, or congestive heart failure, was associated with greater benefit of ACE inhibitors than occurred in lower-risk patients.

The Survival of Myocardial Infarction Long-term Evaluation (SMILE) study used zofenopril beginning within 24 hours after acute anterior MI and continued for 6 weeks. A total of 1,556 patients was randomized to placebo or zofenopril. Within this 6-week interval, ACE inhibitor therapy was associated with a 46% reduction in risk of severe congestive heart failure and a 25% decrease in mortality (absolute reduction, 1.6%; Figure 3-14). In 1 year, absolute mortality reduction in the ACE inhibitor group was >4% lower

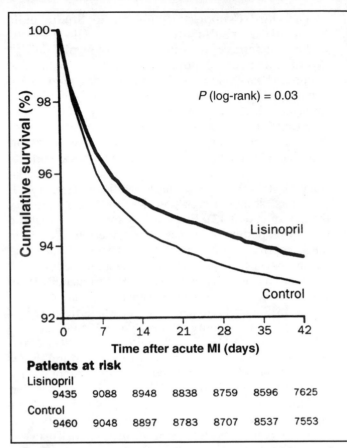

Figure 3-13: Six-week survival in patients treated with lisinopril or nitrates and in the respective control groups in the third Gruppo Italiano per lo Studio della Sopravvivenza nell'Infarto

than in control patients (14.1% vs 10%, relative risk reduction 29%, P <0.011) (Figure 3-15). As in the GISSI-3 trial, much of the decrease in mortality occurred during the early infarct period. At 1 year, 13.1% of the placebo group and

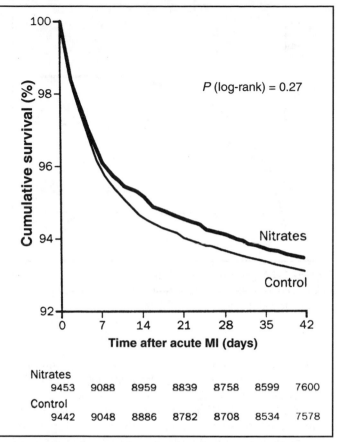

Nitrates						
9453	9088	8959	8839	8758	8599	7600
Control						
9442	9048	8886	8782	8708	8534	7578

Miocardico (GISSI-3) trial. From *Lancet* 1994;343;1115-1122, with permission.

10.4% of the zofenopril patients were taking β-blockers. The target dose of 60 mg daily of zofenopril was achieved in 79% of patients, and adverse effects were observed in 6.8% of the placebo group and 8.6% of zofenopril patients.

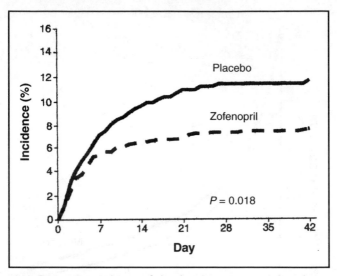

Figure 3-14: Incidence of death or severe congestive heart failure during 6 weeks of treatment with zofenopril or placebo in patients with acute myocardial infarction. From Ambrosioni et al, *N Engl J Med* 1995;332:80-85, with permission.

The effects of acute intervention with ACE inhibitor therapy during thrombolysis in patients with anterior MI were assessed in the Captopril and Thrombolysis Study (CATS). Captopril (Capoten®) 6.25 mg or placebo was administered to 298 patients immediately on completion of intravenous streptokinase (Streptase®). The captopril dose was repeated at 4 and 8 hours and increased to 12.5 mg and 25 mg at 16 and 24 hours, respectively. The target dose was 25 mg t.i.d. At 1 year, there was less LV dilatation and heart failure in the group with combined thrombolysis and captopril than in the thrombolysis-placebo patients (Figure 3-16). It was concluded that very early ACE inhibitor therapy reduced the occurrence of LV dilatation and progression to heart failure.

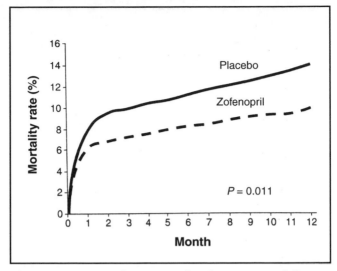

Figure 3-15: Cumulative mortality during 1-year follow-up among patients with acute myocardial infarction treated for 6 weeks with zofenopril or placebo. From Ambrosioni et al, *N Engl J Med* 1995;332:80-85, with permission.

Three major studies assessed the effects of ACE inhibitors early (3 to 16 days) after acute MI in patients with LV dysfunction or heart failure: Survival and Ventricular Enlargement (SAVE), Acute Infarction Ramipril Efficacy (AIRE), and Trandolapril (Mavik®) Cardiac Evaluation (TRACE). Follow-up ranged from 15 months (AIRE) to 50 months (TRACE). The ACE inhibitors were added to diuretics. Mortality was reduced significantly in all three studies: 18% in TRACE, 19% in SAVE, and 27% in AIRE. In AIRE, 2,006 patients were randomized to ramipril (Altace®) or placebo on days 3 to 10 after acute MI. β-Blockers were used in 24% of the ramipril group and 21% of placebo patients. Ramipril reduced the risk of sudden cardiac death by 30%, and the decrease in mortality was apparent at 30 days.

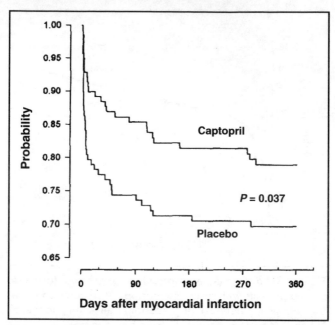

Figure 3-16: Curves representing the absence of heart failure during 1-year follow-up period for captopril-treated patients compared with the placebo group in the Captopril and Thrombolysis Study (CATS). From van Gilst et al, *J Am Coll Cardiol* 1996;28:114-121, with permission.

After an average follow-up of 15 months, in addition to the 27% (*P* <0.002) decrease in all-cause mortality, ramipril produced a 19% (*P* <0.008) reduction in the prespecified end points of cardiac death, heart failure, and stroke. There was no difference in medication withdrawals in the ramipril and placebo groups. A long-term evaluation (42 to 59 months) following the initial AIRE results demonstrated a relative risk reduction of 36% in all-cause mortality (absolute reduction, 11%) in the ACE inhibitor group.

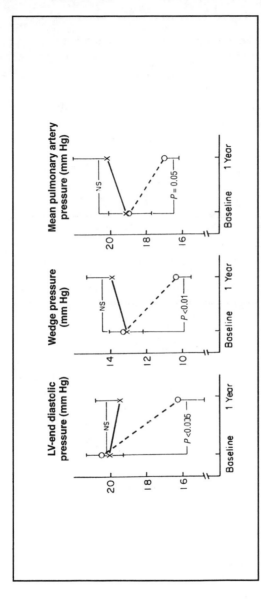

Figure 3-17: Survival and Ventricular Enlargement trial. Change in left ventricular (LV)-end diastolic pressure, pulmonary capillary wedge pressure, and mean pulmonary artery pressure between baseline and 1-year evaluation in the placebo (crosses) and captopril (circles) groups. Values are means ± standard error of mean. No significant difference (NS) between the baseline and one-year values in the placebo group. From Pfeffer et al, *N Engl J Med* 1988;319:80-86, with permission.

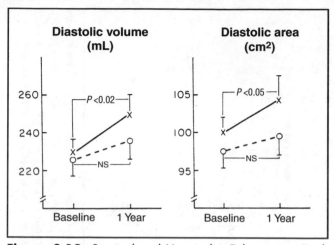

Figure 3-18: Survival and Ventricular Enlargement Trial. Changes in ventricular end diastolic volume and area in the treatment groups (crosses, placebo; circles, captopril). From Pfeffer et al, *N Engl J Med* 1988;319:80-86, with permission.

SAVE (2,231 patients, LV ejection fraction ≤40%) evaluated the effects of captopril administered 3 to 16 days after acute MI with LV dysfunction. The initial dose of captopril, 12.5 mg, was progressively increased to a target of 50 mg t.i.d. and compared to placebo. The beneficial effects of captopril in attenuating hemodynamic dysfunction and ventricular dilatation after 1 year are shown in Figures 3-17 and 3-18. These results were paralleled in the captopril patients by significantly improved clinical outcomes, including reduced cardiovascular mortality and multiple cardiovascular end points (Figure 3-19). After an average follow-up of 42 months, captopril reduced mortality by 19% (P <0.02), new heart failure by 37% (P <0.001), and recurrent MI by 25% (P <0.01).

TRACE included 1,749 patients randomized to trandolapril (up to 4 mg/day) or placebo 3 to 7 days after

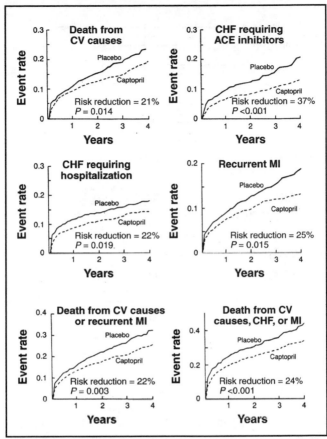

Figure 3-19: Life tables for cumulative fatal and nonfatal cardiovascular (CV) events after recovery from myocardial infarction (MI) in the Survival and Ventricular Enlargement (SAVE) trial. The bottom right panel shows death from CV causes, severe congestive heart failure (CHF) requiring angiotensin-converting enzyme (ACE) inhibitors or hospitalization, or recurrent MI. For the combined analyses, only the time to first event from index infarction used. From Pfeffer et al, *N Engl J Med* 1992;327:669-677, with permission.

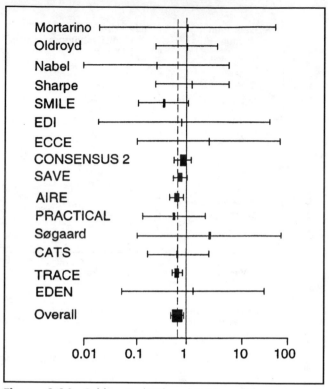

Figure 3-20: Odds ratio (OR) and 95% confidence intervals (CI) for the end point of sudden cardiac death (SCD) in each of 15 trials of angiotensin-converting enzyme (ACE) inhibitors after myocardial infarction. The overall OR for SCD in patients randomized to ACE inhibitors was 0.80 (CI, 0.70 to 0.92). Results are shown on a log scale with box width proportional to the sample size. From Domanski et al, *J Am Coll Cardiol* 1999;33:598-604, with permission.

acute MI with LV dysfunction. Echocardiographically estimated LV ejection fraction ≤35% was an inclusion criterion. There was a significant increase in survival in pa-

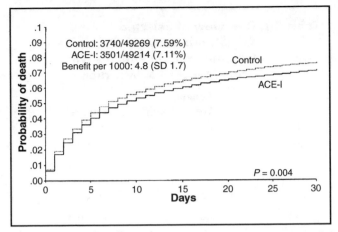

Figure 3-21: The effect of angiotensin-converting enzyme inhibitor (ACE-I) therapy on cumulative mortality during days 0 to 30 in 98,496 patients from four eligible trials of early treatment of ACE-I in acute myocardial infarction: Cooperative New Scandinavian Enalapril Survival Study II (CONSENSUS II), Gruppo Italiano per lo Studio della Sopravvivenza nell'Infarto Miocardico (GISSI-3), Fourth International Study of Infarct Survival (ISIS-4), and Chinese Cardiac Study (CCS-1). From *Circulation* 1998;97:2202-2212, with permission.

tients on trandolapril compared to placebo: 6.2 years vs 4.6 years post-MI, respectively (+27 months, 95% confidence interval 7 to 51). It was also noted that the number of lives saved after 1, 2, and 4 years was 32, 55, and 66 per 1,000 patients treated, respectively.

The composite result of these three trials was a reduction in overall mortality of approximately 20% by ACE inhibitors, with the number of lives saved ranging from 40 to 70 per 1,000 patients treated. A meta-analysis of 15 trials of ACE inhibitor therapy after MI, including more than 15,000 patients, provided strong evidence for ACE inhibitor reduction of sudden cardiac death (Figure 3-20).

Table 3-1: Overview of Selected Angiotensin-converting Enzyme Inhibitor Trials in Patients With Acute Myocardial Infarction

Trial	Patients Treated with ACE Inhibitor*	Control Subjects*
11 small trials	150/2,175 (6.9)	153/2,119 (7.2)
CONSENSUS II	219/3,044 (7.2)	192/3,046 (6.3)
GISSI-3	597/9,435 (6.3)	673/9,460 (7.1)
ISIS-4	2,088/29,028 (7.2)	2,231/29,022 (7.7)
CCS-1	617/6,814 (9.1)	654/6,820 (9.6)
Overview	3,671/50,496 (7.27)	3,903/50,467 (7.73)
		$P = 0.06$

4.6 lives saved per 1,000 patients.
ACE = angiotensin-converting enzyme
*Deaths/treated (%)
Adapted from Latini et al, *Circulation* 1995;92:3132-3137.

A relevant question is which ACE inhibitor to choose. It is probably not advisable to choose an agent that has not demonstrated efficacy in clinical trials because the agents in this class have different half-lives and metabolism. The results of current clinical trials indicate that

ACE inhibitors should be started during the acute phase of MI and maintained indefinitely, at least in patients with objective evidence of LV dysfunction, regardless of whether congestive heart failure is present (Figure 3-21 and Tables 3-1 and 3-2). However, the results of the Heart Outcomes Prevention Evaluation (HOPE) study provide a basis for considering long-term administration of ACE inhibitors to all patients older than 55 years with coronary artery disease.

The results of the HOPE study have an important bearing on the general application of ACE inhibitors in CHD. The study involved 9,297 high-risk men and women older than 55 years and with evidence of vascular disease (cerebral, coronary, or peripheral) or diabetes (patients with diabetes also had one additional risk factor) but no evidence of heart failure or low LVEF. In one arm of the trial, patients were assigned to receive ramipril or placebo for 5 years with evaluation of the primary outcome of MI, stroke, or death from cardiovascular disease. Administration of ACE inhibitors decreased cardiovascular mortality from 8.6% to 6.1%, MI from 12.3% to 9.9%, and stroke from 4.9% to 3.4%. Cardiac arrest, heart failure, and complications of diabetes were also significantly reduced. These differences occurred despite treatment in both groups that included β-blockers (39%), aspirin or other antiplatelet agents (75% to 77%), and lipid-lowering agents (28%). The beneficial effect of ramipril was similar regardless of patient age, gender, antecedent cardiovascular disease, or prior MI. A striking additional finding was the reduction in new-onset diabetes in the ramipril patients. The results support the use of ACE inhibitors in middle-aged men and women with cardiovascular disease or in those at high risk for CHD. Whether to extrapolate these findings to younger patients in these categories must be determined on an individual patient basis. Comparative data on ACE inhibitors regarding dosage and half-life are shown in Table 3-3.

Table 3-2: Summary of Randomized Clinical Trials in High-risk Myocardial Infarction Patients

	SAVE	AIRE	TRACE
Pts randomized	2,231	2,006	1,749
Population	EF ≤40%	CHF	WMI <1.2
Drug initiation from MI (days)	3-16	3-10	3-7
Drug dose (mg)	Cap 12.5 -50 t.i.d.	Ram 2.5 -5 b.i.d.	Tran 1-4
Follow-up (mo)	24-60	6-30	24-50
Mortality (%) Control	24.6	23	62.3
Treated	20.4	17	34.7
Reduction (%)	19	27	18
P	0.019	0.002	0.001
Lives saved/ 1,000/month	1.0	3.5	2.9

EF = ejection fraction; MI = myocardial infarction;
CHF = congestive heart failure; WMI = wall motion index;
Cap = captopril (Capoten®); Ram = ramipril (Altace®);
Zof = zofenopril;
Enal = enalapril (Vasotec®); Tran= trandolapril (Mavik®)

Recently, concern has arisen about a possible adverse interaction between aspirin and ACE inhibitors. The pharmacodynamic effects of ACE inhibitors and aspirin on prostaglandin synthesis are counteractive. This may be especially important in moderate to severe heart failure, in which

SMILE	CATS	CONSENSUS II
1,556	298	6,090
Ant MI	Ant MI	MI
Non-T	T	
≤1	≤6 h	≤1
Zof 7.5 -30	Cap 6.25 -25	Enal 5 -20 b.i.d.
12	3	mean 6
6.5 4.9	4.0 6.0	9.4 10.2
24	—	—
0.198	0	0
11.2	—	—

Adapted from Latini et al, *Circulation* 1995;92: 3132-3137.

prostaglandin synthesis, inhibited by aspirin, may be an important mechanism of vasodilation, potentially enhanced by ACE inhibitors. The Cooperative New Scandinavian Enalapril Survival Study II (CONSENSUS II) trial evaluated early administration of enalapril (Vasotec®) within 24

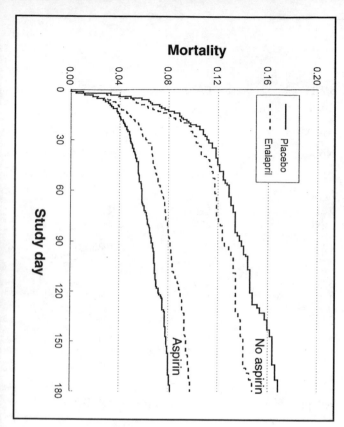

Figure 3-22: Cumulative mortality in the Cooperative New Scandinavian Enalapril Survival Study II (CONSENSUS II) reported in days 0 to 180, stratified by aspirin use at baseline. From Nguyen et al, Am J Cardiol 1997;79:115-119, with permission.

hours of MI and did not show improved survival during 180 days of follow-up (Figure 3-22). A follow-up evaluation of that trial indicated excess mortality when enalapril was randomized to patients using aspirin. By contrast, a meta-analysis of all trials involving more than 1,000 patients randomly allocated to ACE inhibitors early in acute MI and continuing for at least 4 to 6 weeks showed that ACE inhibitor therapy was associated with similar proportional reductions in 30-day mortality compared with controls, regardless of whether aspirin was also administered (Table 3-1). These trials included the Chinese Cardiac Study (CCS-1), CONSENSUS II, GISSI-3, and ISIS-4, totaling more than 96,000 patients, of whom 89% received aspirin. Killip class II or III heart failure was present in 17% of patients in the aspirin group and 26% of patients in the no-aspirin group. The results indicate that, in general, aspirin and ACE inhibitors are both beneficial early in MI. The issue of aspirin/ACE inhibitor interaction is currently under investigation in a prospective, randomized trial.

Angiotensin II Receptor Blockers

While ACE inhibitors block the effects of angiotensin II by reducing its synthesis, angiotensin II receptor blockers (ARBs) provide more specific antagonism by blocking the angiotensin II AT_1 receptor. These agents have not been tested to the extent of ACE inhibitors for efficacy following acute MI, but trials are now under way, and one has been reported. The recently published Optimal Trial in Myocardial Infarction with the Angiotensin II Antagonist Losartan (OPTIMAAL) compared the effects on mortality and morbidity of treatment with losartan (Cozaar®) vs captopril. The trial included more than 5,000 patients with MI and heart failure during the acute phase or a new Q-wave anterior infarction or reinfarction. Losartan was titrated to a target dose of 50 mg once daily, and captopril was titrated to a dose of 50 mg t.i.d., as tolerated. During a mean follow-up interval of 2.7 years, there was a nonsignificant

Table 3-3: Comparative Data on Angiotensin-Converting Enzyme Inhibitors

Drug	Dosing Range (mg)	Target Dose (mg/day)
Benazepril (Lotensin®)	5-40	20
Captopril (Capoten®)	25-50	150
Enalapril (Vasotec®)	5-40	20
Fosinopril (Monopril®)	10-40	20
Lisinopril (Prinivil®, Zestril®)	5-40	20
Moexipril (Univasc®)	7.5-30	15
Perindopril (Aceon®)	4-16	8
Quinapril (Accupril®)	5-80	20
Ramipril (Altace®)	1.25-20	10
Trandolapril (Mavik®)	1-8	4

Adapted from O'Keefe et al, *J Am Coll Cardiol* 2001; 37:1-8.

difference in total mortality favoring captopril (18% vs 16%; relative risk 1.13; $P = 0.07$). There were also no significant differences in the secondary and tertiary cardiac end points of mortality and morbidity. However, losartan therapy was better tolerated than captopril. Therefore, this study supports the primary role of ACE inhibitors in the treatment of post-MI LV dysfunction, with consideration of ARBs when ACE inhibitors are not well tolerated. The Valsartan in Acute Myocardial Infarction (VALIANT) trial compared outcomes after acute MI associated with LV dysfunction or heart failure in patients treated with captopril, valsartan

Half-life (h)	Available Dosage Forms
10-11	5, 10, 20, 40 mg tabs
<2	12.5, 25, 50, 100 mg tabs
11	2.5, 5, 10, 20 mg tabs; 1.25 mg/mL injection
11	10, 20, 40 mg tabs
13	2.5, 5, 10, 20, 40 mg tabs
2-9	7.5, 15 mg tabs
8-10	2, 4, 8 mg tabs
2	5, 10, 20, 40 mg tabs
13-17	1.25, 2.5, 5, 10 mg tabs
16-24	1, 2, 4 mg tabs

(Diovan®), or combination therapy with both agents. The study involved more than 14,000 patients with acute MI. The results were published in the *New England Journal of Medicine* in November 2003 and were important in demonstrating the noninferiority of an ARB compared with an ACE inhibitor for decreasing cardiovascular events in high-risks patients after MI.

VALIANT randomized patients within 10 days of AMI to valsartan, valsartan plus captopril, or captopril. Over a median follow-up of 2 years, no significant differences were seen for the primary end points of overall mortality and the

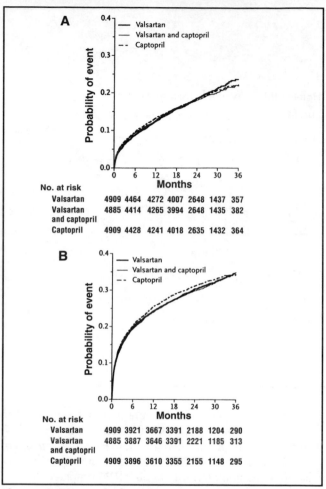

Figure 3-23: Results from the Valsartan in Acute Myocardial Infarction (VALIANT) trial. The end points of death from any cause (A) and combined cardiovascular end point of rate of death from cardiovascular causes, reinfarction, or hospitalization for heart failure (B) outcomes were equal among the three groups. Pfeffer et al, *N Engl J Med* 2003;349:1893-1906, with permission.

Figure 3-24

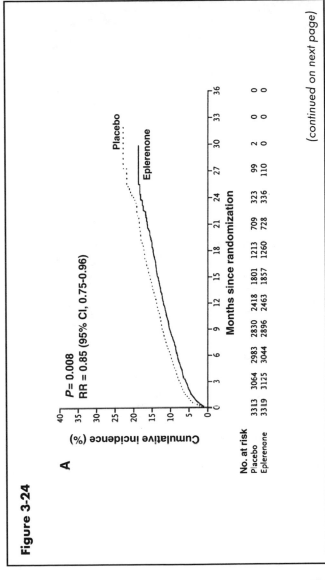

(continued on next page)

121

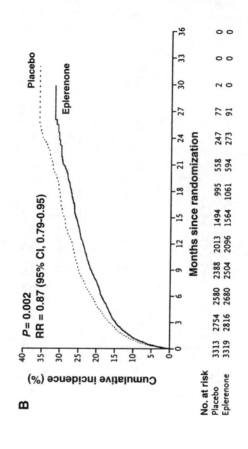

B

Cumulative incidence (%)

P = 0.002
RR = 0.87 (95% CI, 0.79-0.95)

Placebo

Eplerenone

Months since randomization

No. at risk												
Placebo	3313	2754	2580	2388	2013	1494	995	558	247	77	2	0
Eplerenone	3319	2816	2680	2504	2096	1564	1061	594	273	91	0	0

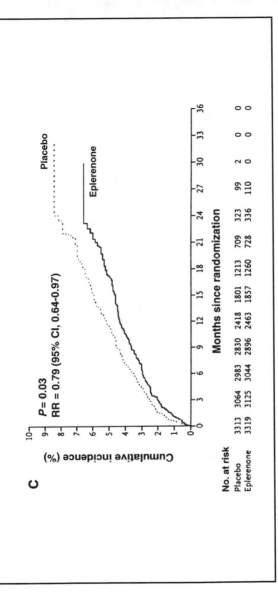

Figure 3-24: Kaplan-Meier estimates of (A) the rate of death from any cause, (B) the rate of death from cardiovascular causes or hospitalization for cardiovascular events, and (C) the rate of sudden death from cardiac causes. The Eplerenone Post-Acute Myocardial Infarction Heart Failure Efficacy and Survival Study (EPHESUS). With permission from Pitt et al, N Engl J Med 2003;348:1309-1321.

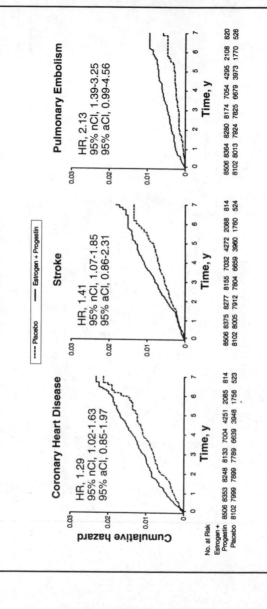

Coronary Heart Disease
HR, 1.29
95% nCI, 1.02-1.63
95% aCI, 0.85-1.97

Stroke
HR, 1.41
95% nCI, 1.07-1.85
95% aCI, 0.86-2.31

Pulmonary Embolism
HR, 2.13
95% nCI, 1.39-3.25
95% aCI, 0.99-4.56

Placebo ---- Estrogen + Progestin ——

Cumulative hazard

Time, y

No. at Risk

Coronary Heart Disease								
Estrogen + Progestin	8506	8353	8248	8133	7004	4251	2085	814
Placebo	8102	7999	7899	7789	6639	3948	1756	523

Stroke								
Estrogen + Progestin	8506	8375	8277	8155	7032	4272	2088	814
Placebo	8102	8005	7912	7804	6659	3960	1760	524

Pulmonary Embolism								
Estrogen + Progestin	8506	8364	8280	8174	7054	4295	2108	820
Placebo	8102	8013	7924	7825	6679	3973	1770	526

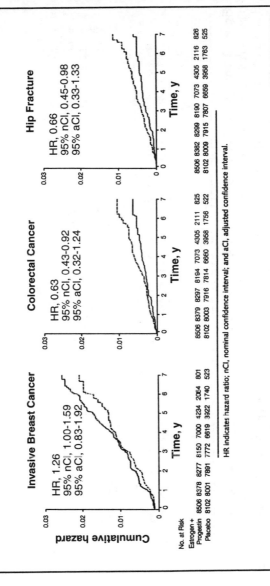

Figure 3-25: Kaplan-Meier estimates of cumulative hazards for selected clinical outcomes in the Heart and Estrogen/Progestin Replacement Study (HERS). From *JAMA* 2002;288:321-333, with permission.

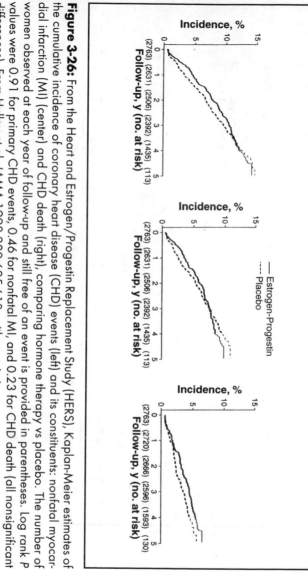

Figure 3-26: From the Heart and Estrogen/Progestin Replacement Study (HERS), Kaplan-Meier estimates of the cumulative incidence of coronary heart disease (CHD) events (left) and its constituents: nonfatal myocardial infarction (MI) (center) and CHD death (right), comparing hormone therapy vs placebo. The number of women observed at each year of follow-up and still free of an event is provided in parentheses. Log rank P values were 0.91 for primary CHD events, 0.46 for nonfatal MI, and 0.23 for CHD death (all nonsignificant differences). From Hulley et al, JAMA 1998;280:605-613, with permission.

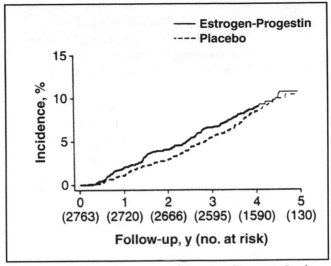

Figure 3-27: From the Heart and Estrogen/Progestin Replacement Study (HERS), Kaplan-Meier estimate of cumulative incidence of death from any cause, hormone therapy vs placebo. The number of women observed at each year of follow-up and still free of an event is provided in parentheses. Log rank *P* value is 0.56 (nonsignificant difference). From Hulley et al, *JAMA* 1998;280:605-613, with permission.

composite end point of fatal and nonfatal cardiovascular events in the three groups (Figure 3-23). For the rate of death from any cause, $P = 0.98$ for valsartan vs captopril and $P = 0.73$ for valsartan + captopril vs captopril. For the rate of death from cardiovascular causes, reinfarction, or hospitalization for heart failure, $P = 0.20$ for valsartan vs captopril and $P = 0.37$ for valsartan + captopril vs captopril. A statistical assessment of noninferiority was used to evaluate the outcomes, demonstrating the statistical significance of the results.

In the OPTIMAAL trial, there had been a strong trend in favor of the ACE inhibitor for death from any cause. However, the ARB dose had not been optimal (losartan

Table 3-4: Overall Relative Hazards of Main Outcomes Comparing Women Randomized to Hormone Therapy With Those Randomized to Placebo

	Unadjusted intention-to-treat
Venous thromboembolism	2.08 (1.28-3.39)
Biliary tract surgery	1.48 (1.12-1.95)
Cancer	
Breast	1.27 (0.84-1.94)
Lung	1.39 (0.84-2.28)
Colon	0.81 (0.46-1.45)
Any	1.19 (0.95-1.50)
Fracture	
Hip	1.61 (0.98-2.66)
Wrist	0.98 (0.64-1.50)
Spine	0.87 (0.52-1.48)
Any	1.04 (0.87-1.25)
Total mortality	1.10 (0.92-1.31)

CI = confidence interval

* Adjusted models are adjusted for age and for predictors of the outcome in a multivariate model at $P < 0.20$ (adjusted treatment effects are similar in larger models that include additional covariates); all covariates are

50 mg/d vs captopril 150 mg/d). The VALIANT trial used optimal doses of the ARB (up to 160 mg/d), thus raising the question of whether higher doses would have increased the effectiveness of losartan in OPTIMAAL.

Hazard Estimate (95% CI)	
Adjusted intention-to-treat*	**Adjusted as-treated****
2.06 (1.26-3.36)	3.04 (1.46-6.31)
1.44 (1.10-1.90)	1.35 (0.94-1.93)
1.27 (0.84-1.94)	1.11 (0.61-2.03)
1.43 (0.87-2.37)	1.73 (0.93-3.21)
0.82 (0.46-1.47)	0.58 (0.25-1.35)
1.19 (0.95-1.50)	1.24 (0.91-1.68)
1.61 (0.97-2.66)	1.18 (0.54-2.58)
1.00 (0.65-1.53)	0.90 (0.54-1.49)
0.89 (0.53-1.50)	0.80 (0.36-1.77)
1.07 (0.89-1.29)	0.97 (0.76-1.23)
1.08 (0.91-1.29)	1.11 (0.84-1.47)

those measured at randomization except for statins, which are current use.
** As-treated analyses were restricted to women who remained adherent to randomly assigned treatment.
From Hulley et al, *JAMA* 2002;288:58-66, with permission.

Angiotensin II receptor blockers appear to have equal efficacy to ACE inhibitors in the treatment of hypertension, and early findings suggest that this is also true for congestive heart failure. However, the recently completed Evaluation of Losartan in the Elderly II (ELITE II) trial involving more than 3,000 patients with congestive heart failure demonstrated that the ARB losartan was better tolerated than the ACE inhibitor captopril, although there was no difference in survival. In small-scale studies, combination therapy with ACE inhibitors and ARBs appears to be superior to ACE inhibitor monotherapy in regard to exercise tolerance, hemodynamic effects, and neurohumoral attenuation. The Randomized Evaluation of Strategies for Left Ventricular Dysfunction (RESOLVD) pilot study indicated superiority of combination therapy in preventing LV dilatation and improving LVEF.

Although the combination of an ACE inhibitor and an ARB may be beneficial in the setting of congestive heart failure or decreased LV function in improving symptoms and hemodynamic function, there is no evidence for improved survival with this approach.

Aldosterone Blockade

Demonstration of the benefits of aldosterone antagonism by spironolactone (Aldactone®) in severe chronic heart failure has led to application of this approach in patients with acute MI complicated by LV dysfunction. In the latter setting, the new selective aldosterone blocker, eplerenone (Inspra®), was evaluated in more than 6,000 patients receiving optimal medical therapy. Eplerenone (25 mg/d initially, titrated to a maximum of 50 mg/d) was initiated 3 to 14 days after acute MI in patients with LVEF ≤40%. As shown in Figure 3-24, eplerenone resulted in significant decreases in all-cause mortality, cardiovascular death or hospitalization for cardiovascular causes, and sudden death during the post-MI period. Severe hyperkalemia occurred in 5.5% of the eplerenone group and 3.9% of placebo patients ($P = 0.002$), while the incidence of hypokalemia in the eplerenone and placebo groups was 8.4% and 13.1%, respectively ($P < 0.001$). This large study

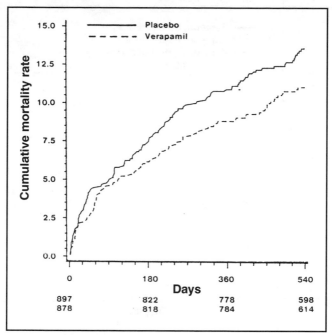

Figure 3-28: Danish Verapamil Infarction Trial (DAVIT II) results. Cumulative mortality rate according to treatment, $P = 0.11$ (not significant). The numbers of patients at risk are shown at the bottom (placebo, n = 897; verapamil, n = 878). From *Am J Cardiol* 1990;66:779-785, with permission.

suggests a role for long-term aldosterone blockade in the management of post-MI patients with LV dysfunction.

Hormone Replacement Therapy

Recent prospective, randomized trials have radically altered the previously favorable view, based solely on retrospective data, of estrogen replacement therapy for secondary prevention of cardiovascular mortality and morbidity. Primary among the controlled trials is Heart and

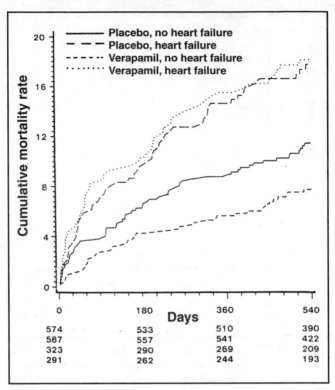

Figure 3-29: Danish Verapamil Infarction Trial (DAVIT II) results. Cumulative mortality rates in patients with heart failure (differences not significant) and without heart failure (P = 0.02), according to treatment. The number of patients at risk are shown at the bottom (placebo, no heart failure, n = 574; verapamil, no heart failure, n = 587; placebo, heart failure n = 323; verapamil heart failure, n = 291). From *Am J Cardiol* 1990;66:779-785, with permission.

Estrogen/Progestin Replacement Study (HERS), published in 1998. HERS was the first prospective, randomized trial to test the concept that HRT conferred beneficial cardiovascular effects in secondary prevention. Based on HERS

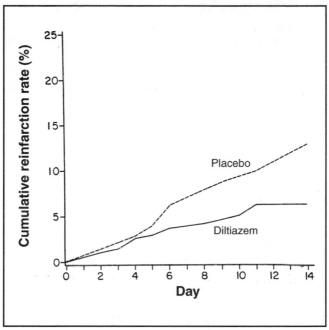

Figure 3-30: Multicenter trial of reinfarction after non-Q-wave infarction. Life-table cumulative reinfarction rates showing significant reduction in reinfarction by the diltiazem group (*P* = 0.03). From Gibson et al, *N Engl J Med* 1986;315:423-429, with permission.

and on other recent studies, a consensus statement by the American Heart Association in 2001 advised against using HRT in women for secondary prevention of cardiovascular disease. The recent results of the Women's Health Initiative primary prevention study indicated small but adverse effects of HRT on cardiovascular events, which indicates a need to broadly reconsider the efficacy of such intervention in regard to cardiovascular risk in general. As shown in Figure 3-25 from the latest study, HRT was

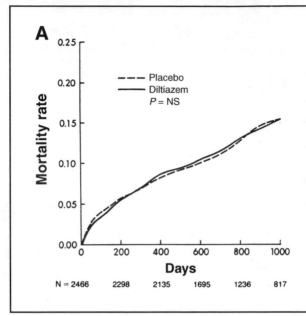

Figure 3-31: Multicenter trial of reinfarction for all infarcts (Q-wave or non-Q-wave). Cumulative rate of total mortality (panel A) and first recurrent cardiac events (panel B), according to treatment. The numbers of patients at risk are

associated with higher rates of CHD, pulmonary embolism, stroke, and breast cancer, whereas the frequency of colorectal cancer and hip fracture was lower.

Estrogen promotes gene expression leading to regulation of vasomotor tone and responses that may inhibit atherosclerosis and ischemia. On the other hand, HRT, frequently a combination of estrogen and progestin (the latter included to minimize the possibility of endometrial cancer in the patient with an intact uterus), has possible prothrombotic and proinflammatory effects. These include increases in factor VII and C-reactive protein and a decrease in anti-

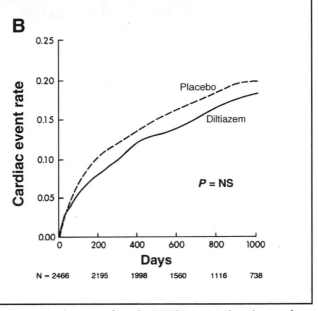

B

shown at the bottom of each panel. In panel B, the reinfarction rate was significantly less with diltiazem at <180 days. NS = not significant. From *N Engl J Med* 1988;319:385-392, with permission.

thrombin III. The beneficial effects of estrogen on the endothelium are presumed to be secondary to the increased synthesis of NO. Other observable benefits of estrogen include decreases in fibrinogen and plasminogen activator inhibitor. It is well established that estrogen increases high-density lipoprotein and decreases low-density lipoprotein concentrations by approximately 10% to 15%. Although estrogen also increases triglyceride levels by approximately 20%, the clinical significance of this finding is unknown.

Previous secondary prevention observational studies of HRT may be marred by selection bias leading to misinter-

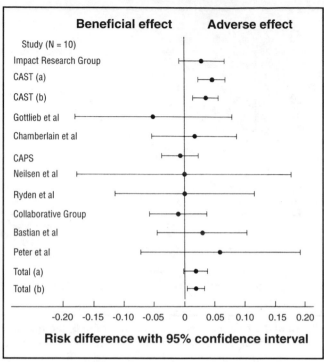

Figure 3-32: Meta-analysis of empirical long-term antiarrhythmic therapy after myocardial infarction. Mean case-fatality rate differences, treated-control for each study and combined. The Cardiac Arrhythmia Suppression Trial (CAST) data are presented twice, based on slight differences in total deaths in analysis of active treatment group. CAPS = Cardiac Arrhythmia Pilot Study. From Hine et al, *JAMA* 1989;262:3037-3040, with permission.

pretation of results. Different characteristics of women who were taking HRT compared with those who were not may have favorably influenced outcomes, independent of HRT. These may include patient age, socioeconomic status, and lifestyle factors, such as smoking, diet, and exercise.

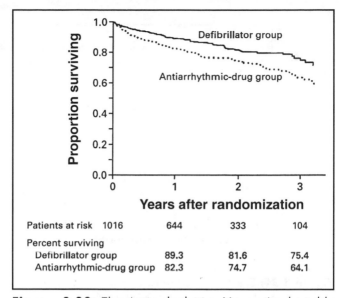

Figure 3-33: The Antiarrhythmics Versus Implantable Defibrillators (AVID) trial. A comparison of antiarrhythmics vs cardioverter-defibrillators in patients resuscitated from near-fatal ventricular fibrillation. Overall survival, unadjusted for baseline characteristics. Survival was better in patients treated with implantable cardioverter-defibrillator (*P* <0.02, adjusted for repeated analyses [n = 6]). From *N Engl J Med* 1997;337: 1576-1583, with permission.

HERS was the first large trial of the effect of postmeno-pausal estrogen plus progestin therapy on the risk for car-diac events. A total of 2,763 women with coronary dis-ease who were postmenopausal with an intact uterus were administered either a combination of conjugated equine estrogen plus medroxyprogesterone or placebo and were followed for more than 4 years. Of these, 17% in each group had previously experienced a Q-wave MI. Although there were no significant differences in the primary out-

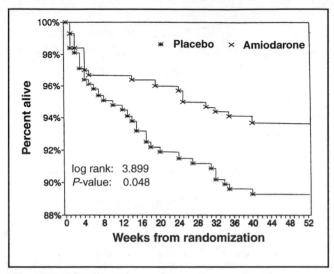

Figure 3-34: Effect of amiodarone on mortality after myocardial infarction. Survival rates of patients who did not die of cardiac causes and were randomly allocated to treatment with amiodarone and placebo during the trial. From Ceremuzynski et al, *J Am Coll Cardiol* 1992;20:1056-1062, with permission.

come of CHD death or nonfatal MI, more CHD events occurred in the first year (especially in the first 4 months) and fewer in the fourth and fifth years in the treatment group compared with placebo (Figures 3-26 and 3-27). Venous thromboembolic disease and gallbladder disease were also more prevalent in the treatment group. The results of this study have been subjected to considerable interpretation and publicity. The possibility of early harm and late benefit could be explained by the initial estrogen effects of thrombogenic and possibly proinflammatory potential outweighing the beneficial effects on lipid levels, antioxidation, and improvement in endothelial function, with a reversal in the later years.

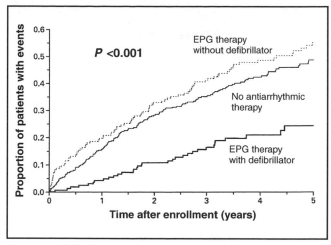

Figure 3-35: Kaplan-Meier estimates of the rates of overall mortality according to whether patients received treatment with a defibrillator in a randomized study of the prevention of sudden cardiac death in patients with coronary artery disease. The P value refers to two comparisons: between the patients in the group assigned to electrophysiologically guided (EPG) therapy who received treatment with a defibrillator and those who did not receive such treatment and between patients assigned to EPG therapy who received treatment and those assigned to no antiarrhythmic therapy. The overall mortality at 5 years was 24% in the defibrillator group and 55% in those who did not receive defibrillators. From Buxton et al, *New Engl J Med* 1999;341:1882-1890, with permission.

HERS-2, a 6.8-year follow-up of the original HERS trial, showed findings similar to those of the original study (Table 3-4). Hormone replacement therapy was associated with small but significant increases in venous thromboembolism and biliary tract surgery and no significant effect on the rates of other major diseases (cardiovascular deaths, all cancers, fractures).

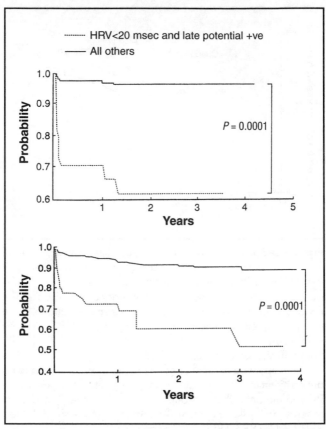

Figure 3-36: Risk stratification for arrhythmic events in postinfarction patients based on heart rate variability (HRV), ambulatory electrocardiographic variables, and the signal-averaged electrocardiogram. Kaplan-Meier survivorship curves are shown for arrhythmic events (top) and cardiac mortality (bottom) in patients with depressed HRV <20 msec and positive (+ve) late potentials and ventricular ectopic beats. The P values refer to differences in event rates between subgroups (log-rank analysis). From Farrell et al, *J Am Coll Cardiol* 1991;18:687-697, with permission.

The recently published Estrogen Replacement and Atherosclerosis in Older Women (ERA) trial of 309 women assigned to estrogen and medroxyprogesterone or placebo (similar to HERS) demonstrated no benefits of HRT on angiographic progression of coronary artery disease over a mean study period of 3.2 years on the basis of serial coronary angiography. Several trials of HRT for secondary prevention are in progress, including Estrogen in the Prevention of Reinfarction (ESPRIT) and a series of angiographic end point studies.

On the basis of current information, it is recommended that HRT not be initiated for secondary prevention of cardiovascular disease. However, for patients with CHD who are already taking HRT, the decision for continuation should be based on established noncoronary benefits, risks, and patient preference. Development of a cardiac event would be a reason for discontinuation of HRT. There appears to be no increase in risk of in-hospital mortality in those women using HRT who develop an initial MI. Future evaluations of HRT after MI include the effects of varied estrogens and progestins and dosage levels, the role of profiling for thrombogenic and proinflammatory genes, and consideration of other established risk factors. At present, HRT should not be considered in the armamentarium of post-MI therapy.

Calcium-Channel Blockers

Three types of agents currently make up the CCB group: dihydropyridines, verapamil (Calan®, Covera-HS®, Isoptin®, Verelan®), and diltiazem (Cardizem®, Dilacor®, Tiazac®). There is evidence of an adverse effect of the short-acting form of nifedipine (Adalat®, Procardia®), particularly at high doses, in patients with ACS and chronic CHD. On the other hand, there is no clear evidence for adverse effects of nondihydropyridines instituted after acute MI. For example, the Danish Study of Verapamil in Myocardial Infarction (DAVIT I and II) resulted in a trend toward benefit in the verapamil groups (Figures 3-28 and 3-29). Diltiazem has

Table 3-5: Comparison of Holter Variables, Late Potentials, Ejection Fraction, and Exercise Test in the Prediction of Arrhythmic Events After Myocardial Infarction

	Sensitivity (%)
Heart rate variability <20 msec	92
Mean relative risk interval <750 msec	67
Late potentials	63
Ventricular ectopic beats <10/h	54
Repetitive ventricular forms	54
Ejection fraction <40%	46
Positive exercise test	50

From Farrell et al, *J Am Coll Cardiol* 1991;18:687-697, with permission.

been extensively evaluated on the basis of the Diltiazem Reinfarction Trial and other multi-institutional studies. Although diltiazem was shown to exert no overall effect on mortality or cardiac events in patients with previous infarction, it was beneficial after non-Q-wave infarctions associated with adequate LV function in preventing severe angina and reinfarction, without effect on mortality (Figure 3-30). However, mortality was increased in patients with depressed LV function. In the results of the long-term Multicenter Diltiazem Postinfarction trial, with follow-up of 25 months, diltiazem reduced the early (<6 months) but not the late (>6 months) rate of reinfarction (Figure 3-31).

More recent studies, especially with long-acting CCBs, have shown no adverse effect on mortality or a slight ben-

Specificity (%)	Positive Predictive Accuracy (%)	Negative Predictive Accuracy (%)
77	17	77
72	13	97
81	17	81
82	16	82
81	15	97
75	10	75
50	6	50

efit. A recent cohort study of more than 11,000 patients with established coronary artery disease (70% with prior MI), receiving nifedipine, verapamil, diltiazem, or placebo, showed no differences in mortality after a mean follow-up period of 3.2 years. In a recently published, community-based registry of MI and cardiac death from the World Health Organization Monitoring Trends and Determinants of Cardiovascular Disease (MONICA) Project, involving almost 4,000 patients with nonfatal suspected MI, no excess risk of recurrent MI or death was found in patients receiving nifedipine, verapamil, or diltiazem compared with patients not receiving CCBs or β-blockers.

In summary, long-acting CCBs can be recommended as adjunctive agents for blood pressure control and de-

Table 3-6: Comparison of Tests for Predicting Major Arrhythmic Events After Myocardial Infarction

Test (No. of Reports)	Number of Patients Studied	Prior Probability (ie, Total MAE Incidence) (Annualized)
ECG-based Tests		
SAECG (22)	9,883	7.99% (4.1%)
SVA (16)	9,564	6.50% (3.33%)
HRV (11)	5,719	9.02% (4.72%)
Left Ventricular Function		
LVEF	7,294	8.57% (4.41%)
Electrophysiologic Studies		
EPS (9)	4,022	8.11% (4.17%)

CI = confidence interval; ECG = electrocardiography; EPS = electrophysiologic study; FN = false negative; FP = false positive; HRV = heart rate variability; LVEF = left ventricular ejection fraction; MAE = major arrhythmic events; SAECG = signal-averaged electro-

Composite Weighted Values for:		2-Year Probability of an MAE if:		Relative Risk	Odds Ratio
Sensitivity (95% CI)	Specificity (95% CI)	Test (+) (95% CI)	Test (-) (95% CI)	(Test +/ Test -)	[(TP/FP)/ (FN/TN)]
62.4% (56.4%- 67.9%)	77.4% (73.6%- 80.8%)	19.3% (18.3%- 20.3%)	4.05% (3.65%- 4.48%)	4.8	5.7
42.8% (32.7%- 53.7%)	80.9% (75.0%- 85.7%)	13.4% (13.0%- 13.7%)	4.68% (4.12%- 5.18%)	2.9	3.2
49.8% (37.5%- 62.1%)	85.8% (82.1%- 88.9%)	25.8% (25.0%- 25.6%)	5.48% (4.37%- 6.52%)	4.7	6.3
59.1% (53.3%- 64.6%)	77.8% (75.5%- 79.9%)	20.0% (19.8%- 19.9%)	4.70% (4.21%- 5.19%)	4.3	5.1
61.6% (48.2%- 73.4%)	84.1% (65.0%- 93.8%)	25.5% (15.6%- 40.7%)	3.88% (3.49%- 4.65%)	6.6	8.5

cardiography; SVA = serious ventricular arrhythmia; TN = true negative; TP = true positive.

From Bailey et al, *J Am Coll Cardiol*, 2001;38:1902-1911, with permission.

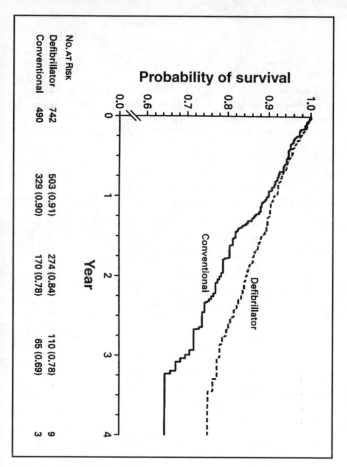

Figure 3-37: Kaplan-Meier estimates of the probability of survival in the group assigned to receive an implantable defibrillator and the group assigned to receive conventional medical therapy in the Multicenter Automatic Defibrillator Implantation Trial II (MADIT II). The difference in survival between the two groups was significant (nominal $P = 0.007$, by the log-rank test). From Moss et al, N Engl J Med 2002;346:877-883, with permission.

Probability of survival

Year

No. at Risk					
Defibrillator	742	503 (0.91)	274 (0.84)	110 (0.78)	9
Conventional	490	329 (0.90)	170 (0.78)	65 (0.69)	3

crease in anginal symptoms in postinfarction patients whose symptoms are not controlled by standard therapy, especially β-blockers. However, CCBs should not be used for cardioprotection.

Nitrates

Except, possibly, for the use of intravenous nitrates during the early acute infarction period, there is variable evidence that prolonged nitrate administration affects survival. The relevance of nitrates after hospital discharge relates to their effect on decreasing ischemic symptoms and their use as an adjunct to hydralazine (Apresoline®) in patients with significant LV dysfunction when ACE inhibitors and ARBs are contraindicated. Their therapeutic efficacy in chronic use has been considered to be related primarily to venodilatation, resulting in decreased preload and, thereby, reduced myocardial oxygen consumption. More recently, large coronary artery dilation has taken on increasing significance as a mechanism of the anti-ischemic action of the nitrates. Large multicenter studies over 4 to 6 weeks following acute MI suggest a decrease in cardiac events during that short period. GISSI-3 and ISIS-4 showed a trend toward overall decrease in cardiac events, although there were no significant effects on cardiac mortality. Because of tolerance to nitrates, a nitrate-free interval is important in their administration. If nitroglycerin patches are used, an 8- to 12-hour drug-free period is necessary. The effective dose varies widely in individual patients. Recommended doses are isosorbide dinitrate 10 to 50 mg q 8 h, transdermal nitroglycerin patch 0.4, 0.8, or 1.2 mg for 12 to 14 hours daily, or isosorbide-5-mononitrate 30 to 120 mg q.d.

Antiarrhythmic Agents

CAST and other relevant studies have demonstrated that the reduction of ventricular ectopy by antiarrhythmic agents may be accompanied by proarrhythmic effects leading to increased mortality and morbidity or, at best, no mortality ben-

147

efit (Figure 3-32). Based on these findings, the routine use of antiarrhythmic drugs post-MI is contraindicated. The main concern raised by postinfarction ventricular dysrhythmias is their significance as a risk factor for sudden cardiac death due to ventricular fibrillation. Of the average 3% to 5% posthospital annual mortality after MI, more than 50% is due to sudden death. (The efficacy of β-blockers in decreasing postinfarction mortality, largely by decreasing the incidence of sudden death, has been considered earlier in this chapter.) Predischarge risk for sudden death has been evaluated by several noninvasively obtained criteria, of which the most widely used have been (1) low LVEF, (2) exercise-induced myocardial ischemia, and (3) frequency of ventricular premature depolarizations. More recently, decreased heart rate variability and abnormal signal-averaged electrocardiography (ECG) (late potentials) have been applied to further identify high risk for sudden death. Those at high risk on the basis of these test findings have usually been treated with an implantable cardioverter-defibrillator (ICD) and/or amiodarone (Cordarone®, Pacerone®) (Figures 3-33, 3-34, and 3-35). The order of most sensitive to least sensitive evaluator for serious dysrhythmias is (1) heart rate variability, (2) late potentials, (3) frequent ventricular ectopic beats, and (4) LVEF <40%. Of these, only heart rate variability has a sensitivity >80% (Figure 3-36, Table 3-5). All four have comparably high specificities. It has been recommended by several authors that, in patients with evidence for ventricular dysrhythmias in the postinfarction state, initial evaluation by signal-averaged ECG and LV ejection be accomplished (Table 3-6). If both tests are positive (ie, positive late potentials are found and LVEF is <40%), the 2-year probability of a serious ventricular dysrhythmia would be >35%, and ICD implantation should be strongly considered. If only one test is positive, ambulatory ECG with a heart rate variability study should be performed. If both of these tests are abnormal (decreased heart rate variability and major ventricular dysrhythmias on ambulatory ECG), ICD implantation should be considered. If only one of these studies is abnormal, electrophysiological testing for vulnerability to life-threatening ventricular dysrhythmias should be performed. This is only one of a number of possible risk stratification pathways. Repetition of this risk stratification can be accomplished at times beyond hospitalization if further evidence of ventricular electrophysiological instability arises.

There is compelling evidence from the recently published Multicenter Automatic Defibrillator Implantation Trial II (MADIT II) (Figure 3-37), together with previous trials, that ICDs improve survival over antiarrhythmic therapy, usually amiodarone, in post-MI patients at high risk for sudden death. High risk in these studies is usually identified by prior MI, reduced LV function (LVEF <30%), and ambient high-grade ventricular ectopy (such as nonsustained ventricular tachycardia). In this setting, ICD implantation has become the therapy of choice.

Conclusions

Based on the considerations discussed and the guidelines for management of patients after acute MI to prevent cardiac mortality, morbidity, and progression of LV dysfunction, the following recommendations are made for patients leaving the hospital after acute MI. Antiplatelet agents, β-blockers, and ACE inhibitors should be administered indefinitely. Antiplatelet dosage should be targeted at 75 to 325 mg/d for aspirin. If aspirin is contraindicated, consider clopidogrel 75 mg/d or warfarin. The international normalized ratio should be kept in the range of 2.0 to 3.0 IU for the latter. Angiotensin-converting enzyme inhibitor dosage should be gradually increased to achieve (1) evidence of LV afterload reduction by lowering systolic blood pressure to <120 mm Hg or (2) a maximum tolerated dose. β-Blockers should be administered in optimal dosage, based on the resting heart rate. It would be advisable to reduce heart rate to <75 beats/minute at rest. Long-acting CCBs may be considered for adjunctive therapy for hypertension if β-blockers and ACE inhibitors do not achieve goal blood pressure. Nitrates are not indicated in patients without angina, but patients should always carry a short-acting nitrate to use if needed. Antiarrhythmic agents are not indicated after uncomplicated MI, but asymptomatic patients at risk for lethal arrhythmias should be considered for an ICD. Once-daily medication will increase patient compliance. Lipid-lowering agents are considered in Chapter 4. Tables 4-5 and 4-6 list current evidence-based American Heart Association/ American College of Cardiology guidelines for comprehensive secondary prevention therapy after acute MI.

Suggested Readings

A comparison of antiarrhythmic-drug therapy with implantable defibrillators in patients resuscitated from near-fatal ventricular arrhythmias. The Antiarrhythmics versus Implantable Defibrillators (AVID) Investigators. *N Engl J Med* 1997;337:1576-1583.

Ambrosioni E, Borghi C, Magnani B: The effect of the angiotensin-converting-enzyme inhibitor zofenopril on mortality and morbidity after anterior myocardial infarction. The Survival of Myocardial Infarction Long-Term Evaluation (SMILE) Study Investigators. *N Engl J Med* 1995;332:80-85.

Bailey JJ, Berson AS, Handelsman H, et al: Utility of current risk stratification tests for predicting major arrhythmic events after myocardial infarction. *J Am Coll Cardiol* 2001;38:1902-1911.

Barron H, Viskin S: Dispelling the myths surrounding the use of beta-blockers in patients after myocardial infarction. *Prev Cardiol* 1998;3:13-15.

Basu S, Senior R, Raval U, et al: Beneficial effects of intravenous and oral carvedilol treatment in acute myocardial infarction. A placebo-controlled, randomized trial. *Circulation* 1997;96:183-191.

Bradley EH, Holmboe ES, Mattera JA, et al: A qualitative study of increasing β-blocker use after myocardial infarction: why do some hospitals succeed? *JAMA* 2001;285:2604-2611.

Braunwald E, Antman EM, Beasley JW, et al: ACC/AHA 2002 guideline update for the management of patients with unstable angina and non-ST-segment elevation myocardial infarction: a report of the American College of Cardiology/American Heart Association Task Force on Practice Guidelines (Committee on the Management of Patients With Unstable Angina). *J Am Coll Cardiol* 2002;40: 1366-1374. Available at: http://www.acc.org/clinical/guidelines/unstable/unstable.pdf. Accessed on May 16, 2003.

Buxton AE, Lee KL, Fisher JD, et al: A randomized study of the prevention of sudden death in patients with coronary artery disease. Multicenter Unsustained Tachycardia Trial Investigators. *N Engl J Med* 1999;341:1882-1890.

Carvedilol Or Metoprolol European Trial. *Lancet* 2003. In press.

Ceremuzynski L, Kleczar E, Krzeminska-Pakula M, et al: Effect of amiodarone on mortality after myocardial infarction: a double-blind, placebo-controlled, pilot study. *J Am Coll Cardiol* 1992;20: 1056-1062.

Chen J, Marciniak TA, Radford MJ, et al: Beta-blocker therapy for secondary prevention of myocardial infarction in elderly diabetic patients. Results from the National Cooperative Cardiovascular Project. *J Am Coll Cardiol* 1999;34:1388-1394.

Dargie HJ: Effect of carvedilol on outcome after myocardial infarction in patients with left-ventricular dysfunction: the CAPRICORN randomised trial. *Lancet* 2001;357:1385-1390.

Dickstein K, Kjekshus J: Effects of losartan and captopril on mortality and morbidity in high-risk patients after acute myocardial infarction: the OPTIMAAL randomised trial. Optimal Trial in Myocardial Infarction with Angiotensin II Antagonist Losartan. *Lancet* 2002;360:752-760.

Domanski MJ, Exner DV, Borkowf CB, et al: Effect of angiotensin converting enzyme inhibition on sudden cardiac death in patients following acute myocardial infarction. A meta-analysis of randomized clinical trials. *J Am Coll Cardiol* 1999;33:598-604.

Effect of ramipril on mortality and morbidity of survivors of acute myocardial infarction with clinical evidence of heart failure. The Acute Infarction Ramipril Efficacy (AIRE) Study Investigators. *Lancet* 1993;342:821-828.

Effect of verapamil on mortality and major events after acute myocardial infarction (the Danish Verapamil Infarction Trial II— DAVIT II) *Am J Cardiol* 1990;66:779-785.

Farrell TG, Bashir Y, Cripps T, et al: Risk stratification for arrhythmic events in postinfarction patients based on heart rate variability, ambulatory electrocardiographic variables and the signal-averaged electrocardiogram. *J Am Coll Cardiol* 1991;18:687-697.

Gheorghiade M, Goldstein S: β-blockers in the post-myocardial infarction patient. *Circulation* 2002;106:394-398.

Gheorghiade M, Schultz L, Tilley B, et al: Effects of propranolol in non-Q-wave acute myocardial infarction in the beta blocker heart attack trial. *Am J Cardiol* 1990;66:129-133.

Gibson RS, Boden WE, Theroux P, et al: Diltiazem and reinfarction in patients with non-Q-wave myocardial infarction. Results of a double-blind, randomized, multicenter trial. *N Engl J Med* 1986; 315:423-429.

GISSI-3: effects of lisinopril and transdermal glyceryl trinitrate singly and together on 6-week mortality and ventricular function after acute myocardial infarction. Gruppo Italiano per lo Studio della Sopravvivenza nell'infarto Miocardico. *Lancet* 1994;343: 1115-1122.

Gottlieb SS, McCarter RJ, Vogel RA: Effect of beta-blockade on mortality among high-risk and low-risk patients after myocardial infarction. *N Engl J Med* 1998;339:489-497.

Hine LK, Laird NM, Hewitt P, et al: Meta-analysis of empirical long-term antiarrhythmic therapy after myocardial infarction. *JAMA* 1989;262:3037-3040.

Hjalmarson A, Herlitz J, Holmberg S, et al: The Goteborg metoprolol trial. Effects on mortality and morbidity in acute myocardial infarction. *Circulation* 1983;67:I26-I32.

Hulley S, Furberg C, Barrett-Connor E, et al: Noncardiovascular disease outcomes during 6.8 years of hormone therapy: Heart and Estrogen/progestin Replacement Study follow-up (HERS II). *JAMA* 2002;288:58-66.

Hulley S, Grady D, Bush T, et al: Randomized trial of estrogen plus progestin for secondary prevention of coronary heart disease in postmenopausal women. Heart and Estrogen/progestin Replacement Study (HERS) Research Group. *JAMA* 1998;280:605-613.

Indications for ACE inhibitors in the early treatment of acute myocardial infarction: systematic overview of individual data from 100,000 patients in randomized trials. ACE Inhibitor Myocardial Infarction Collaborative Group. *Circulation* 1998;97:2202-2212.

Kendall MJ, Lynch KP, Hjalmarson A, et al: Beta-blockers and sudden cardiac death. *Ann Intern Med* 1995;123:358-367.

Latini R, Maggioni AP, Flather M, et al: ACE inhibitor use in patients with myocardial infarction. Summary of evidence from clinical trials. *Circulation* 1995;92:3132-3137.

McCormick D, Gurwitz JH, Lessard D, et al: Use of aspirin, β-blockers, and lipid-lowering medications before recurrent acute myocardial infarction: missed opportunities for prevention? *Arch Intern Med* 1999;159:561-567.

Metoprolol in acute myocardial infarction (MIAMI). A randomised placebo-controlled international trial. The MIAMI Trial Research Group. *Eur Heart J* 1985;6:199-226.

Moser M: Angiotensin-converting enzyme inhibitors, angiotensin II receptor antagonists and calcium channel blocking agents: a review of potential benefits and possible adverse reactions. *J Am Coll Cardiol* 1997;29:1414-1421.

Moss AJ, Zareba W, Hall WJ, et al: Prophylactic implantation of a defibrillator in patients with myocardial infarction and reduced ejection fraction. *N Engl J Med* 2002;346:877-883.

Nguyen KN, Aursnes I, Kjekshus J: Interaction between enalapril and aspirin on mortality after acute myocardial infarction: subgroup analysis of the Cooperative New Scandinavian Enalapril Survival Study II (CONSENSUS II). *Am J Cardiol* 1997;79:115-119.

O'Keefe JH, Wetzel M, Moe RR, et al: Should an angiotensin-converting enzyme inhibitor be standard therapy for patients with atherosclerotic disease? *J Am Coll Cardiol* 2001;37:1-8.

Otterstad JE, Ford I: The effect of carvedilol in patients with impaired left ventricular systolic function following an acute myocardial infarction. How do the treatment effects on total mortality and recurrent myocardial infarction in CAPRICORN compare with previous beta-blocker trials? *Eur J Heart Fail* 2002;4:501-506.

Phillips KA, Shlipak MG, Coxson P, et al: Health and economic benefits of increased β-blocker use following myocardial infarction. *JAMA* 2000;284:2748-2754.

Pfeffer MA, Braunwald E, Moye LA, et al: Effect of captopril on mortality and morbidity in patients with left ventricular dysfunction after myocardial infarction. Results of the survival and ventricular enlargement trial. The SAVE Investigators. *N Engl J Med* 1992;327:669-677.

Pfeffer MA, Lamas GA, Vaughan DE, et al: Effect of captopril on progressive ventricular dilatation after anterior myocardial infarction. *N Engl J Med* 1988;319:80-86.

Pfeffer MA, McMurray JJ, Velazquez EJ, et al: Valsartan, captopril, or both in myocardiol infarction complicated by heart failure, left ventricular dysfunction, or both. *N Engl J Med* 2003;349:1893-1906.

Pitt B, Remme W, Zannad F, et al: Eplerenone, a selective aldosterone blocker, in patients with left ventricular dysfunction after myocardial infarction. *N Engl J Med* 2003;348:1309-1321.

Poole-Wilson PA, Swedberg K, Cleland JG, et al: Comparison of carvedilol and metoprolol on clinical outcomes in patients with chronic heart failure in the Carvedilol Or Metoprolol European Trial (COMET): randomised controlled trial. *Lancet* 2003;362:7-13.

Randomised trial of intravenous streptokinase, oral aspirin, both, or neither among 17,187 cases of suspected acute myocardial infarction: ISIS-2. ISIS-2 (Second International Study of Infarct Survival) Collaborative Group. *Lancet* 1988;2:349-360.

Reikvam A, Kvan E, Aursnes I: Use of cardiovascular drugs after acute myocardial infarction: a marked shift towards evidence-based drug therapy. *Cardiovasc Drugs Ther* 2002;16:451-456.

Rossouw JE, Anderson GL, Prentice RL, et al: Risks and benefits of estrogen plus progestin in healthy postmenopausal women: principal results from the Women's Health Initiative randomized controlled trial. *JAMA* 2002;288:321-333.

Ryan TJ, Antman EM, Brooks NH, et al: ACC/AHA guidelines for the management of patients with acute myocardial infarction: 1999 update: a report of the American College of Cardiology/ American Heart Association Task Force on Practice Guidelines (Committee on Management of Acute Myocardial Infarction). Available at: http://www.acc.org. Accessed on May 16, 2003.

Scrutinio D, Cimminiello C, Marubini E, et al: Ticlopidine versus aspirin after myocardial infarction (STAMI) trial. *J Am Coll Cardiol* 2001;37:1259-1265.

Sharma SK, Kini A, Marmur JD, et al: Cardioprotective effect of prior β-blocker therapy in reducing creatine kinase-MB elevation after coronary intervention. Benefit is extended to improvement in intermediate-term survival. *Circulation* 2000;102:166-172.

The CAPRICORN Investigators. Effect of carvedilol on outcome after myocardial infarction in patients with left-ventricular dysfunction: the CAPRICORN randomized trial. *Lancet* 2002;357:1385-1390.

The effect of diltiazem on mortality and reinfarction after myocardial infarction. The Multicenter Diltiazem Postinfarction Trial Research Group. *N Engl J Med* 1988;319:385-392.

The Lopressor Intervention Trial: multicentre study of metoprolol in survivors of acute myocardial infarction. Lopressor Intervention Trial Research Group. *Eur Heart J* 1987;8:1056-1064.

Timolol-induced reduction in mortality and reinfarction in patients surviving acute myocardial infarction. *N Engl J Med* 1981;304: 801-807.

Van Gilst WH, Kingma JH, Peels KH, et al: Which patient benefits from early angiotensin-converting enzyme inhibition after myocardial infarction? Results of one-year serial echocardiographic follow-up from the Captopril and Thrombolysis Study (CATS). *J Am Coll Cardiol* 1996;28:114-121.

Velazquez EJ, Pfeffer MA, McMurray JV, et al: VALsartan In Acute myocardial iNfarcTion (VALIANT) trial: baseline characteristics in context. *Eur J Heart Fail* 2003;5:537-544.

Viscoli CM, Horwitz RI, Singer BH: Beta-blockers after myocardial infarction: influence of first-year clinical course on long-term effectiveness. *Ann Intern Med* 1993;118:99-105.

Yusuf S, Zhao F, Mehta SR, et al: Effects of clopidogrel in addition to aspirin in patients with acute coronary syndromes without ST-segment elevation. *N Engl J Med* 2001;345:494-502.

Chapter 4

Management of Established and Emerging Coronary Risk Factors

E pidemiologic and clinical evidence demonstrates a clear association between established risk factors and coronary heart disease (CHD) or other atherosclerotic vascular diseases. These risk factors include dyslipidemia, hypertension, cigarette smoking, diabetes, obesity, and a sedentary lifestyle. Risk factor modification in patients with clinical CHD comprises secondary prevention, in contrast to intervention in patients without clinical CHD, termed primary prevention. As indicated in Figure 4-1, the impact of hypercholesterolemia is amplified in patients with clinical CHD compared to those without CHD. This phenomenon is also true of the other established risk factors and provides an important impetus for intensive risk factor management for secondary prevention.

Emerging risk factors that may affect prognosis include oxidative stress, hyperhomocysteinemia, inflammatory factors, and procoagulant substances. Current evidence suggests their role in CHD, but confirmation by further studies is required. Many of these studies are in progress. The current status of cardiovascular risk factors is summarized in Table 4-1, according to the evidence for: (1) the association of the risk factor with ath-

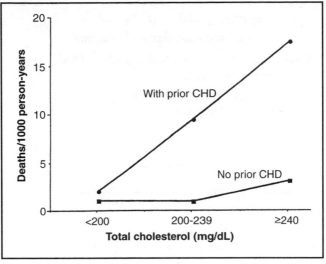

Figure 4-1: Relationship between coronary heart disease (CHD) mortality and total serum cholesterol in populations with and without clinical evidence of prior CHD. From Amsterdam et al, *Am Heart J* 1994;128:1344-1350, with permission.

erosclerotic cardiovascular disease and (2) reduction of the disease by modification of the risk factor.

Lipid Modification

A large number of clinical trials, primarily with HMG-CoA reductase inhibitors (statins), have convincingly demonstrated that lipid lowering significantly reduces coronary artery disease (CAD) mortality and morbidity in patients with CHD, including those who have had a myocardial infarction (MI). A listing of pertinent clinical trials is presented in Table 4-2.

Pathogenic Mechanisms

Lipid abnormalities play a crucial role in the genesis of atheromatous coronary artery plaques. Hyperlipidemia leads to increased platelet reactivity, endothelial dysfunction, and

157

Table 4-1: Classification of Cardiovascular Risk Factors

Established—Modification Reduces Clinical Risk

- Cigarette smoking
- Dyslipidemia (elevated LDL cholesterol, low HDL cholesterol)
- Hypertension
- Diabetes (modification reduces risk of microvascular disease)

Probable or Possible—Intervention Data Lacking

- Obesity
- Physical inactivity
- Small, dense LDL cholesterol particles
- Triglycerides
- Homocysteine
- C-reactive protein
- Oxidative stress
- Lipoprotein (a)
- Psychosocial stress
- Infectious agents

Nonmodifiable

- Age
- Sex
- Family history

HDL = high-density lipoprotein
LDL = low-density lipoprotein

plaque progression and disruption, all of which facilitate coronary occlusion and acute coronary syndromes. Oxidized low-density lipoprotein (LDL) particles are a primary factor in these abnormalities, although decreases in high-density lipoprotein (HDL) particles and very-low-density lipoprotein (VLDL) remnants also contribute to atheromatous plaque formation and propagation. The current National Cholesterol Education Program (NCEP) guidelines recommend a plasma LDL cholesterol (LDL-C) level of <100 mg/dL in patients with atherosclerotic cardiovascular disease. However, endothelial nitric oxide (NO) concentration, necessary for protection against superoxide production, begins to decrease with LDL-C concentrations greater than 40 mg/dL and reaches only approximately 30% of baseline levels at LDL-C concentrations greater than 80 mg/dL (Figure 4-2). In the presence of oxidized LDL-C, NO concentration decreases sharply to 15% of control levels at LDL-C concentrations above 30 mg/dL. Platelet thrombogenic potential is also influenced by LDL-C levels and reversed by statins. Hypercholesterolemia is associated with an increase in thromboxane A_2, a potent platelet activator. Statins reduce thrombus formation in an ex vivo model, largely through antiplatelet activity. Other beneficial effects of statins include a reduction of smooth muscle cell plasminogen activator inhibitor-1 (PAI-1) antigen and an increase in endothelial cell-derived tissue plasminogen activator (tPA), both of which improve thrombolytic balance and may be partially independent of lipid concentration effects.

Evidence exists for other vascular effects of statins with the potential for plaque stabilization, such as an increase in endothelial progenitor cells, which could indicate neovascularization of ischemic tissue; a decrease in matrix metalloproteinases; and fewer macrophages. Studies of leg blood flow have demonstrated an inverse and continuous relationship between plasma cholesterol level and endothelium-dependent dilatation, with no apparent lower threshold (Figure 4-3).

Table 4-2: Overview of Clinical Trials of Lipid Lowering After Myocardial Infarction

Trial	Subjects	MI (mo)*
POSCH** (1990)	838	6-60
4S† (1994)§	4,444	>6
CARE** (1995)	4,159	3-20
LIPID† (1998)	9,014	3-36
VA-HIT† (1999)	2,531	72
L-CAD‡ (2000)	135	6 d
MIRACL† (2001)	2,100	<4 d

POSCH = Program on the Surgical Control of the Hyperlipidemias: partial intestinal bypass; 4S = Scandinavian Simvastatin Survival Study; CARE = Cholesterol and Recurrent Events; VA-HIT = Veterans Affairs High-Density Lipoprotein Cholesterol Intervention Trial; LIPID = Long-term Intervention with Pravastatin in Ischemic Disease; L-CAD = Lipid-Coronary Artery Disease; MIRACL = Myocardial Ischemia Reduction With Aggressive Cholesterol Lowering; MI = myocardial infarction; RR = relative risk

1 = coronary death; 2 = nonfatal MI; 3 = resuscitated cardiac arrest; 4 = worsening of angina requiring hospitalization; 5 = angiographic progression of

Benefits of Lipid Lowering

Meta-analysis of clinical trials has amply demonstrated the efficacy of statins in reducing LDL-C levels. A 10% reduction of serum cholesterol is associated with a 15%

Time from Follow-up (y)	Mean/Median Findings**
9.7	[1+2] 35% lower
5.4	[1+2+3] RR 0.66
5	[1+2] 24% lower
6.1	[1] 24% lower
5.1	[1+2] 4% lower
2	[5] 42% lower
16 wk	[1+2+3+4] 16% lower

coronary atherosclerosis; combined total mortality, cardiovascular death, nonfatal MI, percutaneous coronary intervention/coronary artery bypass grafting, stroke, new onset peripheral vascular disease; [a+b+c] = combined components for outcome data.

* = Time from coronary event

** = Outcomes in treatment group vs control group

† = MI or unstable angina

‡ = MI and/or percutaneous transluminal coronary angioplasty secondary to unstable angina

§ = Year of publication of major results

From Harjai, *Ann Intern Med* 1999;131:376-386, with permission.

reduction in CHD mortality and an 11% reduction in total mortality risk. Several observational studies have also demonstrated the efficacy of early initiation of statin therapy after MI. In the study of the Swedish Registry of Cardiac

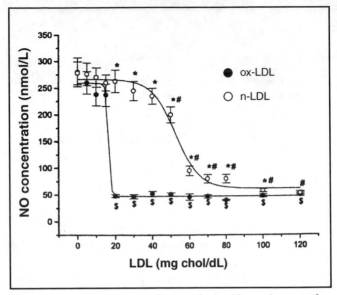

Figure 4-2: Changes in nitric oxide (NO) production after endothelial cells were exposed to native low-density lipoprotein (n-LDL) and oxidized low-density lipoprotein (ox-LDL). Stimulated peak NO concentrations are shown as changes from respective baseline values. Data are expressed as mean ± standard deviation. # = P <0.005 n-LDL vs control; $ = P <0.005 ox-LDL vs control; chol = cholesterol. From Vergnani et al, *Circulation* 2000;101:1261-1266, with permission.

Intensive Care of almost 20,000 patients, statin treatment initiated by hospital discharge was associated with a mortality of 4.0% (unadjusted) at 1 year compared to 9.3% (unadjusted) in patients discharged without a statin (relative risk reduction, 0.75; P = 0.001). Adjusted data indicated a 20% relative reduction in mortality. Lipid measurements were not part of the compulsory data evaluation, but the guidelines for statin intervention were total cholesterol (TC) >200 mg/dL or LDL-C >115 mg/dL. In the Global Use of

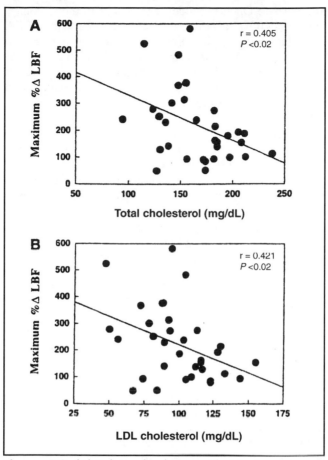

Figure 4-3: (A) Relationship between the maximum percent increments (%Δ) in leg blood flow (LBF) above baseline in response to graded intrafemoral artery infusions of methacholine chloride (MCh) and total cholesterol levels. (B) Relationship between the maximum percent increments in LBF above baseline in response to intrafemoral artery infusions of MCh and low-density lipoprotein (LDL) cholesterol levels. From Steinberg et al, *Circulation* 1997;96:3287-3293, with permission.

Strategies to Open Occluded Arteries in Acute Coronary Syndromes (GUSTO IIb) and Platelet Glycoprotein IIb/IIIA in Unstable Angina: Receptor Suppression Using Integrilin Therapy (PURSUIT) trials involving more than 20,000 patients, the odds of dying at 6 months were 33% lower in patients on lipid-lowering agents, with a 20% reduction in the composite outcome of death or nonfatal MI (both results significant). Mortality reduction began at as early as 30 days in the lipid intervention group.

A recently reported trial of lipid lowering in secondary prevention further indicates the general protective effect of lipid lowering. The Heart Protection Study evaluated 20,536 adults with coronary disease, other occlusive arterial disease, or diabetes, randomized to simvastatin (Zocor®) or placebo. After 5 years of follow-up, the statin group demonstrated a reduction in all-cause mortality of 13%, CHD mortality of 18%, nonfatal MI of 27%, and revascularization and stroke of 25% (Figure 4-4). Among the unique and important aspects of this study was confirmation that statin therapy similarly reduced cardiovascular end points in the entire group of patients, regardless of whether initial baseline LDL-C was $\geq$100 mg/dL or <100 mg/dL. This study provides powerful evidence that lowering LDL-C beyond the current therapeutic target (<100 mg/dL) is beneficial in secondary prevention.

Important post-MI lipid-lowering trials with statins include the Scandinavian Simvastatin Survival Study (4S), the Cholesterol and Recurrent Events (CARE) trial, the Long-term Intervention with Pravastatin in Ischemic Disease (LIPID) study, and the Myocardial Ischemia Reduction with Aggressive Cholesterol Lowering (MIRACL) trial. The first three trials followed patients with MI or unstable angina, with randomization beginning at least 3 months after the acute event. The MIRACL trial randomized patients within days after the acute event. The 4S involved 4,444 patients with angina pectoris (21%) and/or previous MI (79%) and elevated cholesterol levels followed for 5.4 years

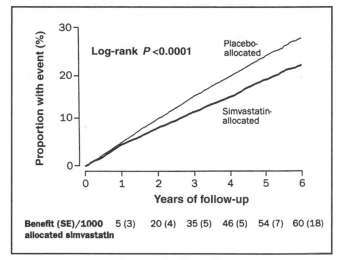

Figure 4-4: Life-table plot of effect of simvastatin allocation on percentages having major vascular events in the Heart Protection Study. From *Lancet* 2002;360:7-22, with permission.

after randomization to simvastatin or placebo. The average LDL-C was 188 mg/dL. In the treatment group, TC decreased by 25%, LDL-C decreased by 35%, and HDL cholesterol (HDL-C) increased by 8%. Nonfatal MI and CHD deaths decreased by 34% in the treatment group. All-cause mortality decreased by 30% (Figures 4-5 and 4-6). A post hoc analysis found that patients with elevated LDL-C, low HDL-C, and elevated triglycerides were more likely to have an increased risk for CHD events on placebo and greater benefit from statin therapy than patients with isolated LDL-C elevation (Figure 4-7).

In the CARE study, 4,159 patients who had a previous acute MI were randomized to pravastatin (Pravachol®) or placebo and followed for 5 years. The average LDL-C was lower than in 4S (range 115 to 174 mg/dL). In the treatment group, TC decreased by 20%, LDL-C decreased

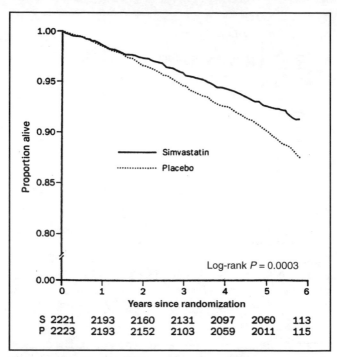

Figure 4-5: Kaplan-Meier curves for all-cause mortality in the Scandinavian Simvastatin Survival Study (4S). Number of patients at risk at the beginning of each year is shown below the horizontal axis. S = simvastatin, P = placebo. From *Lancet* 1994;344:1383-1389, with permission.

by 28%, and HDL-C increased by 5%. Nonfatal MI and CHD deaths decreased by 24% in the treatment group (Figures 4-8 and 4-9). All-cause mortality decreased by 8%. Elderly patients showed a significant benefit of statins (decrease in coronary death from 10.3% to 5.8% and decrease in stroke incidence from 7.3% to 4.5%, compared with placebo; Figures 4-10 and 4-11). Analysis of events in relation to LDL-C levels achieved in both the treatment and placebo groups indicated a reduction in coronary events to a level of 125 mg/dL, but no further benefit was seen below this level. The percentage or absolute reduction of LDL-C, however, had little relationship to events (Figure 4-12). The LIPID trial followed 9,014 patients with acute MI (64%) or unstable angina. In the pravastatin-treated patients, TC decreased by 18%, LDL-C decreased by 25%, and HDL-C increased by 5%. In the statin-treated group, nonfatal MI and CHD death declined by 24%, and all-cause mortality decreased by 22% (Figures 4-13 and 4-14).

All three large, randomized trials demonstrated beneficial effects on primary end points associated with reductions of LDL-C and modest increases in HDL-C. The results of CARE, LIPID, and a primary prevention trial, the West of Scotland Coronary Prevention Study (WOSCOPS), all of which used pravastatin, were pooled to provide enough power to assess specific coronary events. This included 19,768 patients and allowed for the evaluation of 2,194 primary end points. Relative risk reduction was similar throughout most of the baseline LDL-C range (125 to 212 mg/dL), with the possible exception of the lowest quintile of the two secondary prevention studies (<125 mg/dL). Relative risk reduction in the treatment group was significantly decreased irrespective of age, gender, smoking history, and diabetes or hypertension status. Pooled analysis of CARE and LIPID demonstrated a reduction of 22% in coronary death and nonfatal infarction (95% confidence interval, 7% to 34%; $P = 0.005$) (Figures 4-15 and 4-16). There was no significant decrease in event rate for patients with LDL-C <125 mg/dL at baseline.

The most recent large secondary prevention trial with a statin is the GREACE Study (GREek Atorvastatin and Coronary-heart-disease Evaluation Study). Patients with established CHD were randomized to atorvastatin (Lipitor®) (10 to 80 mg/d, n = 800) titrated to achieve LDL-C <100 mg/dL or to usual care (n = 800). During a follow-up

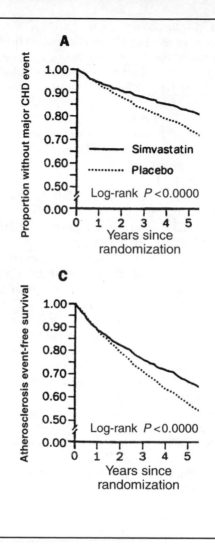

Figure 4-6: Kaplan-Meier curves for secondary and tertiary end points in the Scandinavian Simvastatin Survival Study (4S). (A) Major coronary events; (B) any coronary event; (C) sur-

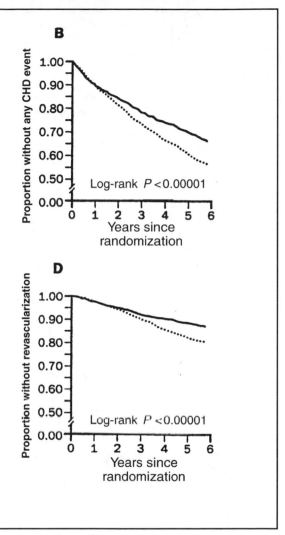

vival free of any atherosclerotic event; (D) myocardial revascularization procedures. From *Lancet* 1994;344:1383-1389, with permission.

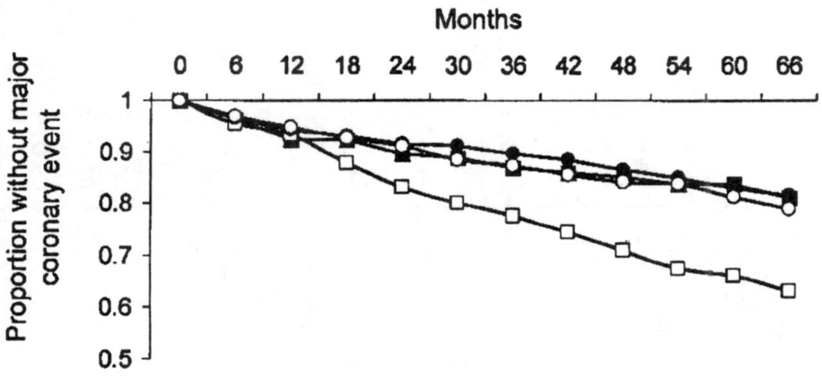

Figure 4-7: Effect of simvastatin on event-free survival by subgroups in the Scandinavian Simvastatin Survival Study (4S), defined by baseline high-density lipoprotein cholesterol (HDL-C) and triglyceride. Event-free survival was significantly lower in patients with combined abnormalities of increased low-density lipoprotein cholesterol (LDL-C), increased triglyceride, and reduced HDL-C ("lipid triad") who received placebo (□) than in other treatment subgroups and improved more with simvastatin in the lipid triad subgroup (■) than the subgroup with isolated LDL-C elevation (●, simvastatin; ○, placebo). From Ballantyne et al, *Circulation* 2001;104:3046-3051, with permission.

period of 3 years, the mean dose of atorvastatin was 24 mg/d, and hyperlipidemia therapy was administered to 14% of the usual-care group. Atorvastatin reduced TC by 36%, LDL-C by 46%, and triglycerides by 31%; HDL-C was raised by 7%. LDL-C <100 mg/dL was achieved in 95% (n = 759) of the atorvastatin group and in 3% of the usual-care patients. During the study, fatal or nonfatal coronary events occurred in 12% of the atorvastatin patients and 24.5% of the usual-care group (risk ratio 0.49, confidence interval 0.27-0.73, P <0.0001). The reductions in primary end points (43% to 59%) produced by atorvastatin are depicted in Figure 4-17. The cost per quality-adjusted life-year gained with atorvastatin was $8,350. Five patients taking atorvastatin were withdrawn from the study because of adverse effects, none of which included myalgia.

In contrast with these studies, the MIRACL trial started intensive statin treatment soon after an acute coronary event (24 to 96 hours). A total of 3,086 patients with unstable angina or non-Q-wave MI (53%/54% MI in treatment/placebo groups) who were not candidates for acute coronary revascularization was randomized to high-dose (80 mg) atorvastatin or placebo with evaluation of outcome over the next 16 weeks. The initial LDL-C levels were modestly elevated (124 mg/dL in both groups). The primary combined end point of death, nonfatal MI, cardiac arrest with resuscitation, or recurrent symptomatic myocardial ischemia requiring rehospitalization was 17.4% in the placebo group and 14.8% in the treatment group (P = 0.048) (Figure 4-18). In terms of individual group outcomes, only the symptomatic ischemia group showed a significant benefit of statin therapy. The changes in lipid levels in the atorvastatin group are of particular interest. The LDL-C values decreased from 124 mg/dL at baseline to 72 mg/dL at the end of the study. Triglycerides fell from 184 mg/dL to 139 mg/dL, and HDL-C increased modestly from 36 mg/dL to 38 mg/dL. The inci-

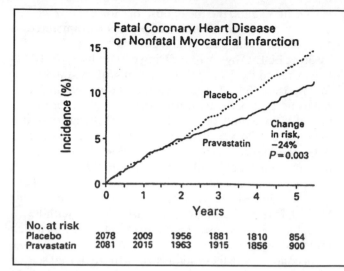

Figure 4-8: Kaplan-Meier estimates of the incidence of coronary events in the pravastatin and placebo groups of the Cholesterol and Recurrent Events (CARE) study. The left-hand panel shows data for the primary end point of fatal coronary heart disease or nonfatal myocardial infarction. The right-hand panel

dence of adverse hepatic effects was 2.5% in the treatment group, which reversed with discontinuation of treatment.

Interestingly, MIRACL demonstrated a significant decrease in stroke in the treatment group (1.6% vs 0.8%), although the incidence was quite low. The high dose of atorvastatin was generally well tolerated, with a serious effect rate of <1% (not significant compared with controls). Although the results did not show a benefit on mortality within this short period, morbidity was significantly reduced. A substantial percentage of patients in each group was on angiotensin-converting enzyme (ACE) inhibitors (49%) and β-blockers (78%), which would tend to minimize the effects of another potential risk-reducing agent. Finally, the largest acceptable dose of the most potent statin

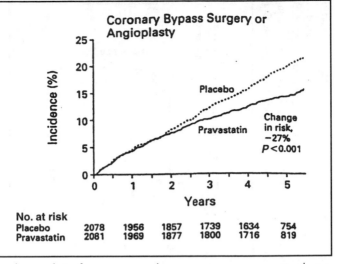

Coronary Bypass Surgery or Angioplasty

No. at risk						
Placebo	2078	1956	1857	1739	1634	754
Pravastatin	2081	1969	1877	1800	1716	819

shows data for coronary bypass surgery or angioplasty. Changes in risk are those attributable to pravastatin. *P* values and changes in risk are based on Cox proportional hazards analysis. From Sacks et al, *N Engl J Med* 1996;335:1001-1009, with permission.

was administered and tolerated. It is possible that a similar effect could be achieved with lower doses. This theory is being subjected to further clinical trials.

Evidence from 4S, CARE, and the Air Force/Texas Coronary Atherosclerosis Prevention Study (AFCAPS/ TexCAPS) shows significant benefits of risk reduction aimed at decreasing LDL-C, even with low HDL-C levels. The ratio of TC/HDL-C may be used to guide therapy, in that very high risk individuals should have a ratio <4, and high-risk individuals should have a ratio <5. In a study of 3,090 patients with either prior MI (78%) or angina, with triglycerides ≤300 mg/dL, and with low HDL-C (≤45 mg/dL), treatment with bezafibrate or placebo yielded no significant difference in primary end points (fatal MI, non-

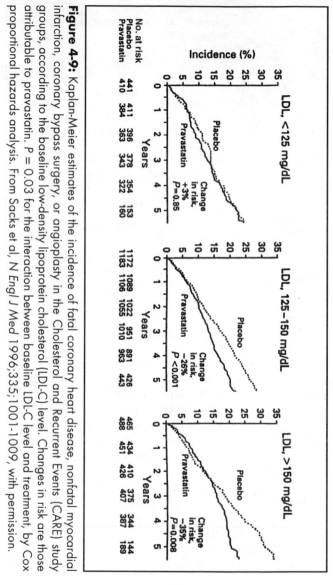

Figure 4.9: Kaplan-Meier estimates of the incidence of fatal coronary heart disease, nonfatal myocardial infarction, coronary bypass surgery, or angioplasty in the Cholesterol and Recurrent Events (CARE) study groups, according to the baseline low-density lipoprotein cholesterol (LDL-C) level. Changes in risk are those attributable to pravastatin. $P = 0.03$ for the interaction between baseline LDL-C level and treatment, by Cox proportional hazards analysis. From Sacks et al, N Engl J Med 1996;335;1001-1009, with permission.

174

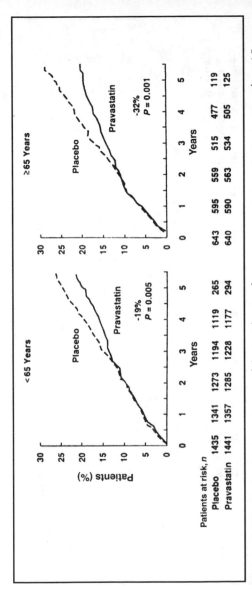

Figure 4-10: Kaplan-Meier estimates of the incidence of coronary events in patients younger than 65 years (left) and aged 65 to 75 years (right) in the Cholesterol and Recurrent Events (CARE) trial. Coronary events are fatal coronary heart disease, nonfatal myocardial infarction, coronary artery bypass grafting, and angioplasty. The percentage relative risk reductions attributable to pravastatin are given above the *P* values. *P* values and risk reduction are based on Cox proportional hazards analysis. From Lewis et al, *Ann Intern Med* 1998;129:681-689, with permission.

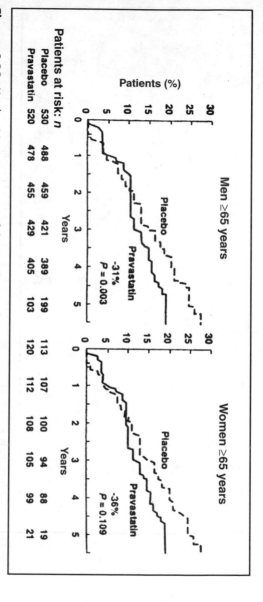

Figure 4-11: Kaplan-Meier estimates of the incidence of coronary events in men (left) and women (right) aged at least 65 years in the Cholesterol and Recurrent Events (CARE) trial. Coronary events are as described in Figure 4-10. The percentage relative risk reductions attributable to pravastatin are given above the P values. Calculations of P values and risk reduction are as indicated in Figure 4-9. From Lewis et al, *Ann Intern Med* 1998;129:681-689, with permission.

fatal MI, or sudden death) after 6.2 years, although HDL-C was increased by 19% and triglycerides were reduced by 21%. In the subgroup with triglyceride levels ≥200 mg/dL, however, the reduction in cumulative probability of a primary event with the fibrate was 40% ($P = 0.02$) (Figures 4-19 and 4-20). In the LIPID trial, statins were just as effective in decreasing mortality in patients with high initial triglyceride levels. It is generally recommended that, with LDL-C >130 mg/dL and triglycerides <500 mg/dL, statins are the first choice in secondary prevention, primarily to reduce LDL-C, but also because of their evident beneficial effects on HDL-C and triglycerides. Fibric acids may be reserved as initial therapy for situations in which LDL-C is <100 mg/dL, HDL-C is <40 mg/dL, and triglyceride level is >200 mg/dL, along with aggressive dietary intervention.

Patterns (1998-1999) for use of lipid-lowering medications in patients at hospital discharge after MI were assessed by Fonarow et al. Less than one third of patients received treatment with these agents (Figure 4-21). In patients with previous CHD, coronary revascularization, or diabetes, the proportion was higher but still less than 50%. Factors that correlated with the use of lipid-lowering agents included a history of elevated cholesterol, cardiac catheterization during hospitalization, smoking cessation counseling, use of a β-blocker, and care in a teaching hospital.

Relevant clinical trials under way include the Treating to New Targets (TNT) Study, the Study of the Effectiveness of Additional Reductions in Cholesterol and Homocysteine (SEARCH), and the Incremental Decrease in Endpoints through Aggressive Lipid lowering (IDEAL) trial. These trials deal mostly with post-MI patients and involve from 8,000 to more than 20,000 patients each. They are mostly 5-year follow-up studies evaluating primary end points of CHD, death, or nonfatal MI. Among the issues being evaluated is the relative efficacy of low-dose vs high-dose statins.

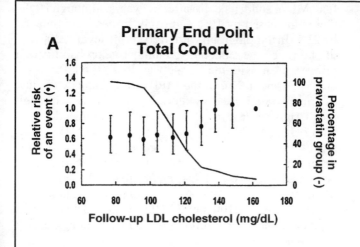

Figure 4-12: Low-density lipoprotein cholesterol (LDL-C) concentration during follow-up and coronary events in the Cholesterol and Recurrent Events (CARE) trial. Placebo and pravastatin groups combined = 4,159 patients. (A) Primary end point: coronary death or nonfatal myocardial infarction (MI) (n = 486 patients with end point, 55 in the 10th decile); (B) expanded end point: coronary death, nonfatal MI, coronary artery bypass graft,

The most recently developed HMG Co-A reductase inhibitor is rosuvastatin (Crestor®), approved in September 2003. Clinical data indicate that it is more potent in lowering LDL-C than any of the currently available statins. Pooled results from three trials that included patients with and without CHD and compared rosuvastatin (10 mg) with atorvastatin (10 mg) have been evaluated. As indicated in Figure 4-22, significantly more patients reached their LDL-C goal with rosuvastatin than with atorvastatin (76% vs 53%, $P <0.001$). Further, the differences in goal achievement were greatest in patients with CAD, in whom the LDL-C goal was <100 mg/dL. In this group, the 10-mg dose of rosuvastatin resulted in

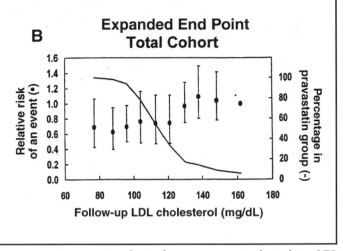

Expanded End Point Total Cohort

or percutaneous transluminal coronary angioplasty (n = 979 patients with end point, 111 in 10th decile). Data points show relative risks with 95% confidence intervals for coronary events for deciles of follow-up LDL concentration. Percentage of patients in each decile of LDL concentration in pravastatin group is indicated by the solid line, corresponding to right vertical axis. From Sacks et al, *Circulation* 1998;97:1446-1452, with permission.

achievement of goal in 60% of patients compared to only 19% of patients taking 10 mg of atorvastatin.

Another recent addition to the lipid-lowering armamentarium is ezetimibe (Zetia®). This agent is the first of a new class of drugs that inhibit the intestinal absorption of cholesterol. It is administered in pill form at a dose of 10 mg/d. In one study, the administration of ezetimibe with a statin provided an incremental 14% decrease in LDL-C, a 5% increase in HDL-C, and a 10% decrease in triglycerides. Lipid-lowering agents in development include bile acid transport inhibitors and inhibitors of acyl CoA:cholesterol acyltransferase.

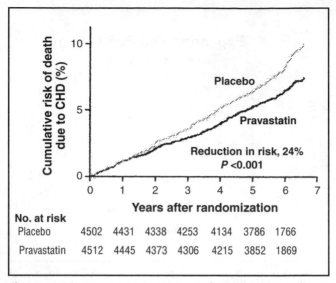

Figure 4-13: Long-term Intervention with Pravastatin in Ischemic Disease (LIPID) study results. Kaplan-Meier estimates of mortality due to coronary heart disease (CHD), the primary outcome, in the pravastatin and placebo groups. Relative reduction of risk was based on Cox proportional hazards model. The P value was based on the log-rank test, with stratification according to the qualifying event. It was estimated that for every 1,000 patients assigned to pravastatin, death from CHD was avoided in 19 patients. From *N Engl J Med* 1998;339:1349-1357, with permission.

Diet and Institutional Issues

Although guidelines for secondary prevention include the implementation of the NCEP Adult Treatment Panel (ATP) III Therapeutic Lifestyle Changes (TLC) diet recommendations—which limit fats to <30% calories, cholesterol to <200 mg, and saturated fats to <7% daily—there is little evidence that this diet is aggressively pursued during hospitalization for MI or after discharge. Issues of nutritional compliance are important. Physicians are generally uncomfortable dealing with nutrition, nutritionists are not usually available in clinical practices, and patient compliance, especially with relatively stringent diets, is low. Nonetheless, there is ample evidence that dietary interventions provide significant risk benefit, especially in secondary prevention.

An example is the Ornish study, involving 48 patients with moderate to severe CAD randomized to intensive lifestyle change vs usual care. The intensive diet consisted of a 10% fat whole foods vegetarian diet, aerobic exercise, stress management training, smoking cessation, and group support for a 5-year period. Coronary arteriograms were evaluated serially. The severity of coronary stenoses decreased in the intensive-treatment group, but increased in the usual-care group. Cardiac events were lower in the intensive-treatment group (risk ratio for control group was 2.5). However, it is highly unlikely that such a regimen could be implemented or followed in an average population compared with this well-motivated volunteer group.

The Mediterranean diet emphasizes more grains, fruit, root and green vegetables, and fish and poultry and less beef, lamb, and pork. Butter is replaced with margarine high in α-linolenic acid. Based on the results of the Lyon Diet Heart Study, the Lyon diet was important, aside from the results, in specifying the form and types of fat-containing foods and oils. The study evaluated 423 post-MI patients randomized to a Mediterranean-type diet or usual diet. The Lyon diet consisted of 30% fat calories, similar to the American Heart Association (AHA) diet, which is based on the NCEP ATP III recommendations. Saturated fat percentage was also similar (8%), but polyunsaturated fatty acids were lower (<5% vs 7% to 10%) with a cholesterol intake equivalent to the TLC diet (<200 mg). After a mean of 46 months' follow-up, the composite outcome of cardiac stroke and nonfatal MI was reduced (14 events in experimental group, 44 in control group) (Figure 4-23). Major secondary end points, such as stroke, angina, or heart

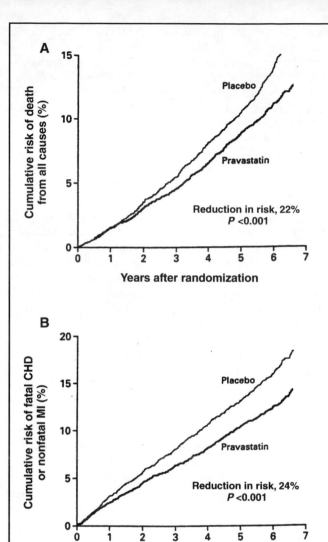

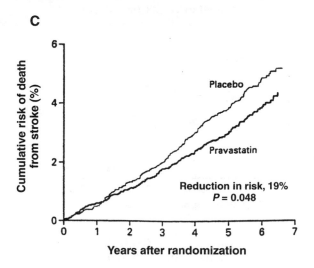

Figure 4-14: Long-term Intervention with Pravastatin in Ischemic Disease (LIPID) study results. Kaplan-Meier estimates of the incidence of major secondary outcomes in the pravastatin and placebo groups. (A) Mortality from all causes; (B) death due to coronary heart disease (CHD) or nonfatal myocardial infarction (MI); and (C) stroke of any type. On the basis of differences in proportions of patients with an event during the entire study period, for every 1,000 patients assigned to pravastatin, death from any cause was avoided in 30 patients, death due to CHD or nonfatal MI was avoided in 35 patients, and stroke was avoided in 8 patients. From *N Engl J Med* 1998;339:1349-1357, with permission.

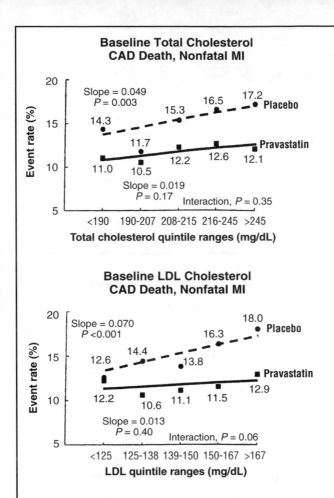

Figure 4-15: Prospective Pravastatin Pooling Project. Coronary event rates according to total and low-density lipoprotein cholesterol (LDL-C) concentrations. Cholesterol and Recurrent Events (CARE) and Long-term Intervention with Pravastatin in Ischemic Disease (LIPID) studies combined, n = 13,173. Lipid distributions were divided into quintiles. Lines are best-fit linear

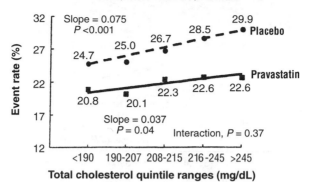

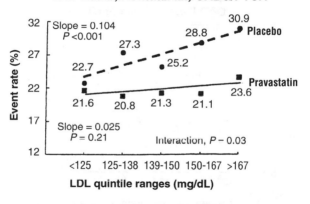

regressions with entire range of plasma total-cholesterol and LDL-C concentrations. 'Interaction' *P* value denotes statistical significance level for test for a relationship between baseline total cholesterol or LDL-C and a reduction in coronary event rates. From Sacks et al, *Circulation* 2000;102:1893-1900, with permission.

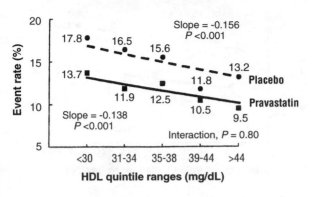

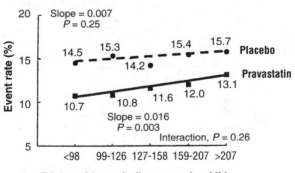

Figure 4-16: Prospective Pravastatin Pooling Project. Coronary event rates according to high-density lipoprotein (HDL) cholesterol and triglyceride concentrations. Cholesterol and Recurrent Events (CARE) and Long-term Intervention with Pra-

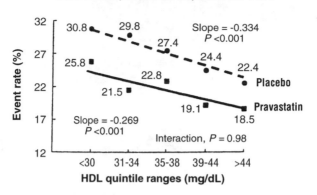

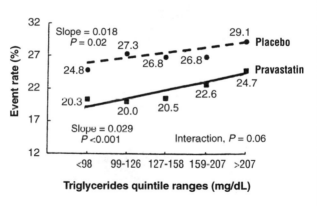

vastatin in Ischemic Disease (LIPID) studies combined, n = 13,173. Statistical analysis methods are the same as in Figure 4-15. From Sacks et al, *Circulation* 2000;102:1893-1900, with permission.

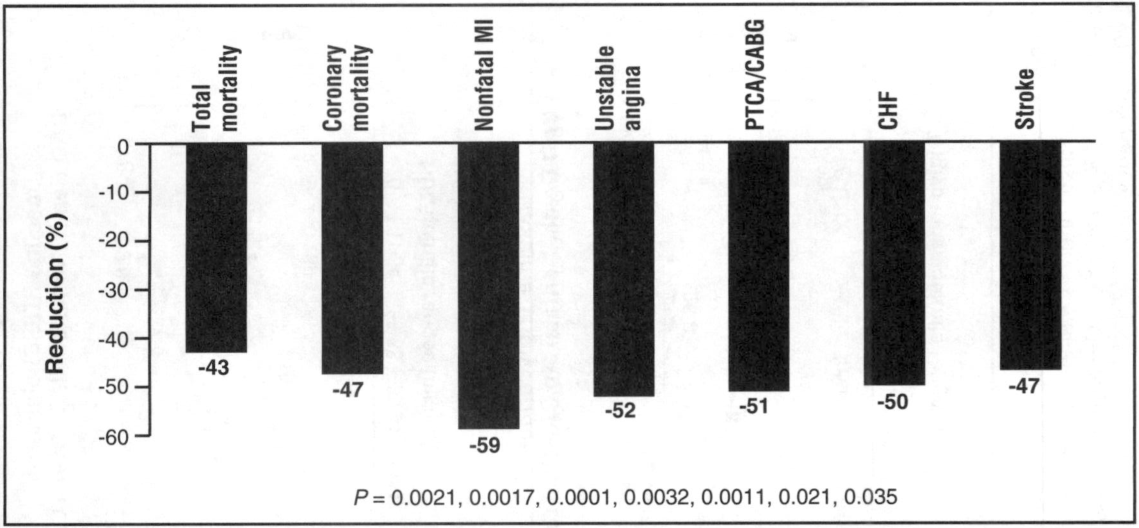

Figure 4-17: Reduction in relative risk of primary end points with atorvastatin in the GREek Atorvastatin and Coronary-heart-disease Evaluation (GREACE) Study. CABG = coronary artery bypass graft, CHF = congestive heart failure, PTCA = percutaneous transluminal coronary angioplasty. With permission from Mikhailidis et al, *Curr Med Res Opin* 2002;18:215-219.

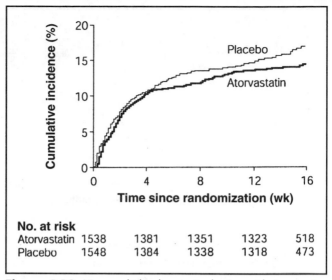

Figure 4-18: Myocardial Ischemia Reduction with Aggressive Cholesterol Lowering (MIRACL) study. Kaplan-Meier estimates of primary outcomes. The relative risk of the composite outcome in the atorvastatin group compared with placebo was 0.84 (95% confidence interval, 0.70 to 1.00; $P = 0.048$) based on Cox proportional hazards analysis. The decrease in number at risk at 16 weeks reflects the fact that many patients completed the study within the days immediately preceding 16 weeks. From Schwartz et al, *JAMA* 2001;285:1711-1718, with permission.

failure, were also significantly reduced in the experimental group (Figure 4-24). Major traditional risk factors, such as cholesterol levels and hypertension, were independent predictors of outcome events.

The results of the Lyon Diet Heart Study have engendered considerable interest. The key points are:

(1) ω-3 Polyunsaturated fatty acids were important in the beneficial outcomes of this study. The ω-3 fatty acids (fish oils) have demonstrated cardioprotective effects, in-

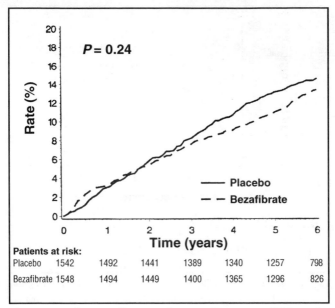

Figure 4-19: Bezafibrate Infarction Prevention (BIP) study. Kaplan-Meier curves for the cumulative probability of the primary event. There was no significant difference. From *Circulation* 2000;102:21-27, with permission.

cluding decreased dysrhythmias, anti-inflammatory properties, decreased synthesis of cytokines, stimulation of endothelium-derived NO, decreased thrombosis tendency, and inhibition of atherosclerosis.

(2) A 50% to 70% reduction in cardiac end points was noted in the intervention group.

(3) Enhanced definition of the baseline diets of both control and intervention groups is important in analysis. The control group did not have this baseline analysis and was assumed to have a diet equivalent to the treatment group.

(4) Potential geographic and nonmeasured cultural and social differences among treatment populations

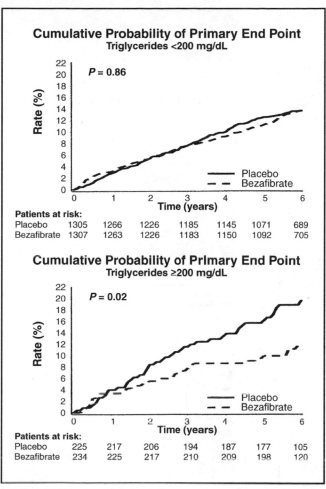

Figure 4-20: Bezafibrate Infarction Prevention (BIP) study. Kaplan-Meier curves for the primary end point in subgroups of patients with baseline triglycerides ≥200 mg/dL and <200 mg/dL. Only in the high baseline triglyceride subgroup were the differences in treatment groups significant. From *Circulation* 2000;102:21-27, with permission.

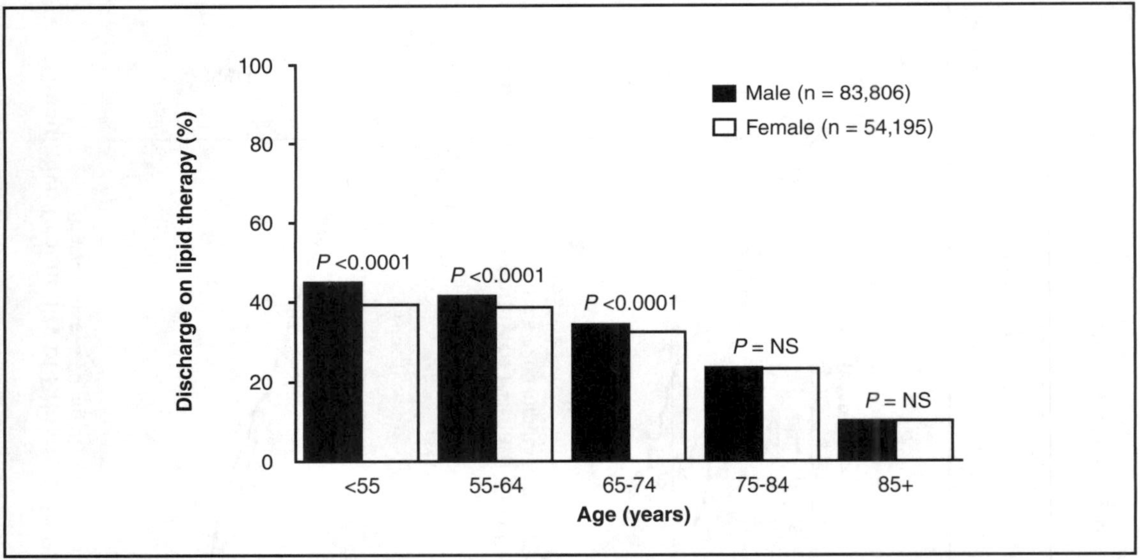

Figure 4-21: From the National Registry of Myocardial Infarction 3. Association of patient age and sex with prescription of lipid-lowering medications at hospital discharge for acute myocardial infarction. From Fonarow et al, *Circulation* 2001;103:38-44, with permission.

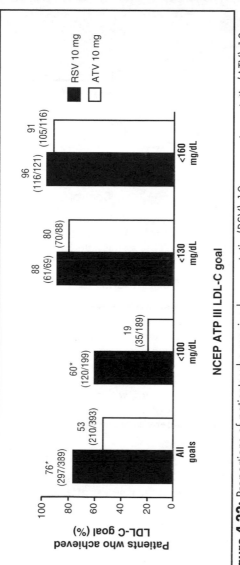

Figure 4-22: Proportions of patients who received rosuvastatin (RSV) 10 mg or atorvastatin (ATV) 10 mg and achieved National Cholesterol Education Program Adult Treatment Panel III (NCEP ATP III) low-density lipoprotein cholesterol (LDL-C) goals at 12 weeks (all goals and by individual goal) based on pooled data from three trials. * *P* <0.001 vs ATV. Numbers in parentheses are number achieving goal/total number in each category. Mean baseline LDL-C levels were 186 mg/dL for RSV 10 mg and 187 mg/dL for ATV 10 mg. From Shepherd et al, *Am J Cardiol* 2003;91:11C-17C.

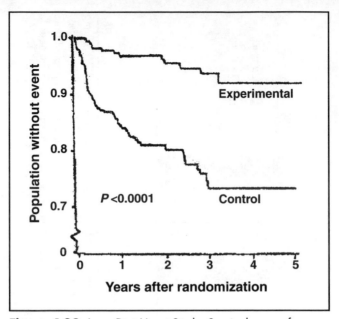

Figure 4-23: Lyon Diet Heart Study. Survival curves for combined cardiac death, nonfatal infarction, unstable angina, heart failure, stroke, and thromboembolism. Log-rank test using the time of the first event was used to compare the control and study (experimental) groups. There was already a striking difference between the two groups within the first year (*P* <0.0001). From De Lorgeril et al, *J Am Coll Cardiol* 1996;28:1103-1108, with permission.

should be assessed in recommending dietary guidelines. In comparison, the TLC diet, although indicating an increase in polyunsaturated fatty acids, makes no additional recommendation to lower the intake of the ω-6 class of essential fatty acids (linolenic acid), which is high in vegetable oils, nor to increase intake of ω-3 fatty acids (α-linolenic acid), found in a few vegetable oils such as canola oil, soybean oil, and flaxseed oil.

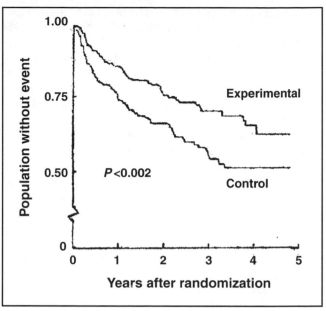

Figure 4-24: Lyon Diet Heart Study. Survival curves for combined major primary and secondary end points and minor end points, including episodes of stable angina necessitating hospital admission, need for elective myocardial revascularization, postangioplasty restenosis, and venous thrombophlebitis. Although statistically significant ($P = 0.0018$), the difference between groups shown here was less impressive than that shown when fewer events were included in the analysis (Figure 4-23). From De Lorgeril et al, *J Am Coll Cardiol* 1996;28:1103-1108, with permission.

There is also no comment about the ω-3 fish oils in the TLC diet.

Trans-fatty acids, formed by partial hydrogenation of vegetable oils, have been associated with increased risk for MI. *Trans*-fatty acids constitute 10% to 60% of total fat in margarine and more than 10% of fat in cookies, crackers, French-fried potatoes, glazed doughnuts, and bread. Although investigators agree that *trans*-fatty acids have adverse effects on cholesterol profiles, there is little agreement on the significance of the problem. Food labeling tends to hide the presence of *trans*-fatty acids because they are incorporated under polyunsaturated and monounsaturated fatty acids. *Trans*-fatty acids can be reduced relatively easily by food manufacturers, but substitution of saturated fatty acids should, of course, be avoided.

There is also evidence that the type of protein ingested may beneficially affect cholesterol levels. A meta-analysis of 38 studies on the effects of soy (vegetable) protein intake on serum lipids demonstrated a significant decrease in LDL-C and triglycerides. The effect was strongly related to the initial cholesterol level. It is possible that the beneficial effects on lipids may be the result of isoflavones or phytoestrogens. A recent scientific conference on dietary fatty acids and cardiovascular health provided a concise series of recommendations on this issue. These included efforts by the food industry to genetically modify crops to produce vegetable oils that contain no saturated fat and *trans*-fatty acid-free products. Examples include soybean and canola oils that provide long-chain ω-3 fatty acids. The result could be more heart-healthy products with little essential dietary changes by consumers.

With regard to soy protein, in 1999, the US Food and Drug Administration (FDA) approved a health claim that an intake of 25 g/d of soy protein reduces the risk for heart disease.

Stanol/sterol ester-containing foods (called 'nutraceuticals') are emphasized in the NCEP III guidelines for cholesterol management. These components are isolated from soybean oils and esterified to increase solubility. Intakes of 2 to 3 g/d of plant sterols may reduce LDL-C by 10% to 20%, although the effect is inconsistent among individuals. There is little effect on HDL-C or triglycerides. These guidelines recommend that the stanol group be reserved for secondary prevention after an atherosclerotic event.

Antioxidants and Homocysteine Reduction

Considerable interest has been generated about the use of antioxidant vitamins because of evidence that superoxide radicals propagate endothelial damage and lead to atheromatous degeneration and plaque breakdown in the arterial wall. Much of the data on the efficacy of such vitamin supplementation is tenuous. However, a large body of literature has developed on the subject, and it is appropriate to review some highlights in reference to secondary prevention strategies.

The specific vitamins at issue are vitamin E and folic acid. The former has antioxidant properties; the latter decreases homocysteine levels. Because elevated homocysteine levels are a risk factor for coronary events, it seems logical to attempt to lower these levels, which can be accomplished by folic acid, with the support of vitamins B_6 and B_{12}.

Vitamin E (α-Tocopherol)

Several well-designed, epidemiologic studies have demonstrated that high vitamin E consumption is associated with a lower cardiovascular risk. However, randomized, prospective clinical trials have yielded inconsistent results. The Cambridge Heart Antioxidant Study (CHAOS), a randomized, controlled trial of vitamin E in patients with coronary disease, evaluated 2,002 patients with angiographic evidence of CAD to determine the efficacy of high doses of vitamin E in reducing the risk for MI. Over approximately 1.5 years, active treatment significantly reduced the risk of cardiovascular death and nonfatal MI (relative risk, 0.53; 95% confidence interval, 0.34 to 0.83). Other studies, notably the Gruppo Italiano per lo Studio della Sopravvivenza nell'Infarto miocardico (GISSI) prevention study, did not demonstrate a significant benefit.

The Heart Outcomes Prevention Evaluation (HOPE) trial, involving subjects at high risk for coronary events, found no efficacy for vitamin E. Moreover, a 3-year trial of 160 patients with CAD and low HDL-C who were randomly assigned to receive antioxidants with lipid-lowering agents demonstrated an attenuation of the protective effect of lipid-lowering therapy when concurrent antioxidants were used (vitamin E, vitamin C, β-carotene, and selenium) (Figure 4-25). In addition, serial coronary angiographic studies indicated that concurrent antioxidants did not significantly attenuate plaque formation, as opposed to the beneficial effect of the lipid-lowering agents alone.

Folic Acid

Folic acid, vitamin B_6, and vitamin B_{12} serve as cofactors in the enzymatic pathways of homocysteine metabolism. Deficiencies of these cofactors increase homocysteine levels. There is strong evidence that increased homocysteine increases the risk for coronary events and predicts mortality, independent of traditional risk factors in CAD patients (Figure 4-26). There is also evidence for the beneficial effects of folate on coronary atherosclerosis (Figure 4-27). Although 'normal' homocysteine plasma levels are <15 µmol/L, the primary cardiovascular risk gradient extends below this level. Elevated homocysteine levels have also been associated with increased ischemic myocardial injury in acute coronary syndromes, on the basis of peak cardiac troponin T levels. In summary, beneficial effects on endothelial function and coronary stenosis have been demonstrated with folate administration in CHD patients. There are no substantive data for decrease in CHD risk with folate administration in hyperhomocysteinemia because the clinical trials have not yet been accomplished. Although folic acid supplementation up to 5 mg/d has been used in patients with high homocysteine levels (>15 µg/L) with the expectation that coronary risk will be reduced, there is, as yet, no strong evidence of a reduction in nonfatal infarction or cardiac death from this intervention. Nonetheless, it may be prudent to administer folate supplementation in doses of 400 µg to 5 mg in post-MI patients with elevated homocysteine levels. It has been found that a dose of 400 μg/d minimizes plasma homocysteine levels in most people. Because the average folate intake in the United States is 200 μg/d, it may be worthwhile to recommend consumption of foods fortified with folate (such as cereals), as has been recommended by the FDA. Indeed, cereals with fortified folate content (500 to 665 μg/serving) have resulted in increases in folate levels of 65% to 106% and decreases in plasma homocysteine of 11% to 14%.

Hypertension, Diabetes, and Smoking

Hypertension, diabetes, and smoking play large roles in primary and secondary CHD events. The 2001 AHA/American College of Cardiology (ACC) guidelines for secondary prevention are succinct about these three risk factors. The diabetes management goal consists of an HbA_{1c} value <7%, using appropriate hypoglycemic agents and lifestyle modification to help maintain this goal, such as weight management and physical activity. For smoking, the goal is obviously complete cessation using available means, including counseling, nicotine replacement, and bupropion (Zyban®).

Hypertension and Left Ventricular Hypertrophy

The *Seventh Report of the Joint National Committee on Prevention, Detection, Evaluation, and Treatment of High Blood Pressure* provides the following key recommendations for patients with CHD. Blood pressure goal is <140/90 mm Hg. Patients with diabetes or chronic kidney disease should have a target goal of <130/80 mm Hg. The first drugs of choice are usually β-blockers (nonintrinsic sympathomimetic) and ACE inhibitors. An aldosterone antagonist and/or a thiazide diuretic is also recommended. Alternatively, long-acting calcium-channel blockers can be used. Short-acting calcium-channel blockers should be avoided. Nondihydropyridines (verapamil [Calan®, Covera®, Isoptin®, Verelan®] and diltiazem [Cardizem®, Cartia®, Dilacor®, Diltia®, Tiazac®]) have been advocated for hypertension with non-Q-wave MI. The use of calcium-channel antagonists is

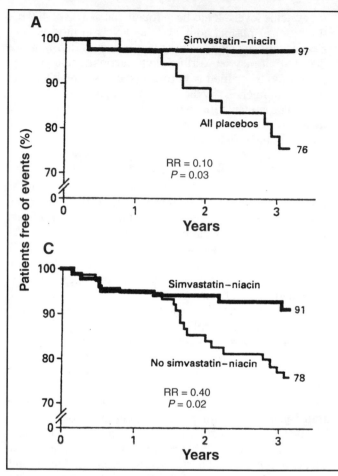

Figure 4-25: Kaplan-Meier curves for the time to the first component of the composite primary end point (death from coronary causes, nonfatal myocardial infarction, confirmed stroke, or revascularization for worsening ischemia) in a 3-year randomized trial. (A) Curves for the 38 patients in the simvastatin-niacin group and for the 38 in the placebo group; the relative risk (RR) for an event was 0.10 (95% confidence intervals, 0.01

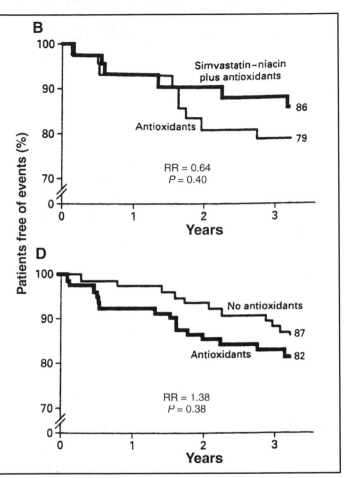

to 0.81). (B) Curves for the 42 patients assigned to receive simvastatin and antioxidants and for the 42 in the antioxidant group. (C) Curves for all 80 patients who were assigned to receive simvastatin plus niacin and for the 80 who were not. (D) Curves for the 84 patients who were assigned to receive antioxidants and for the 76 who were not. From Brown et al, *N Engl J Med* 2001;345:1583-1592, with permission.

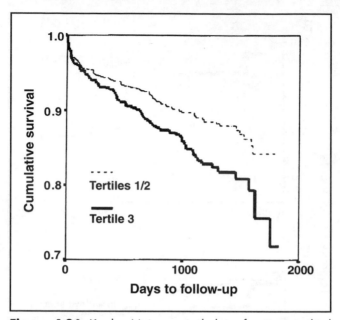

Figure 4-26: Kaplan-Meier survival plots of patients in third homocysteine level (16.2 µg/dL) compared with the first and second tertiles of homocysteine plasma levels from 1,412 patients with severe coronary artery disease. Survival is significantly better in patients in tertiles 1 and 2 (log-rank statistic 10.1, P = 0.0014). From Anderson et al, *Circulation* 2000;102:1227-1232, with permission.

reviewed in Chapter 3. It should also be noted that the ACC/AHA 2002 guidelines for management of unstable angina and non-ST-segment elevation MI recommend a general target blood pressure of no more than <135/85 mm Hg for all patients with acute coronary syndromes.

Whether lowering blood pressure well below 140/90 mm Hg would be beneficial in patients after MI is not known. The Hypertension Optimal Treatment (HOT) study, in which 8% of patients had CHD and <2% had

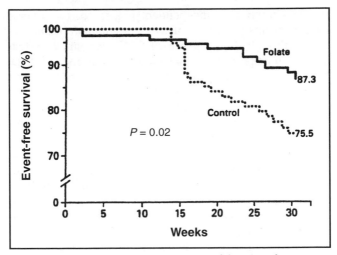

Figure 4-27: Kaplan-Meier analysis of freedom from major adverse cardiac events in 196 patients after successful coronary angioplasty. The rate of event-free survival was significantly higher among patients assigned to folate treatment than among control patients. The relative risk of a major cardiac event with folate treatment was 0.52 (95% confidence interval, 0.28 to 0.98). Revascularization of the target lesion (relative risk, 0.48; 95% confidence interval, 0.25 to 0.94) accounted for most of the observed events described as major. From Schnyder et al, *N Engl J Med* 2001;345:1593-1600, with permission.

previous MI, demonstrated no adverse effects and, in fact, a decrease in adverse cardiac events when diastolic blood pressure had decreased to a mean of 83 mm Hg. However, the small percentage of patients with prior MI in this group precludes extrapolation of the results to MI patients in general.

Another concern is the effect of left ventricular hypertrophy (LVH) on prognosis. A substantial proportion of patients with hypertension (20% to 30%) have echocardiographic evidence for LVH. Left ventricular hypertrophy is a significant, independent risk factor for adverse cardiac events regardless of whether a patient has had an MI. Although the presence of LVH appears to affect women more profoundly than men in the absence of CAD, there is no definitive information on the gender-related impact of differences in LVH in MI patients. It has been demonstrated that hypertension with LVH is associated with coronary vascular remodeling and attenuated endothelial and nonendothelial coronary flow reserve.

Based on these considerations, we recommend the initial use of β-blockers as antihypertensive agents after MI, with appropriate conjunctive use of ACE inhibitors. If either of these classes is contraindicated, we would administer long-acting calcium-channel blockers instead of β-blockers. Whether to use a dihydropyridine or a nondihydropyridine should be determined by factors such as the patient's baseline heart rate. Angiotensin II receptor blockers could be substituted for ACE inhibitors if side effect issues arise. If there is additional evidence for congestive heart failure (CHF) or poor left ventricular ejection fraction and the blood pressure remains elevated, efforts should be made to carefully optimize blood pressure levels to <130/85 to decrease myocardial oxygen needs by decreasing afterload. Thiazide diuretics are usually more effective than loop diuretics in reducing blood pressure, but, if creatinine levels are >2.0 or if significant CHF is present, a loop diuretic would be a better choice. Of course, salt restriction to <6 g/d is important in hypertension, regardless of whether CHF is present.

Diabetes

Type 2 diabetes, which accounts for 85% of diabetes cases, is an important risk factor for CHD, stroke, and peripheral vascular disease. The occurrence of MI in patients with diabetes is often associated with subtle symptoms, frequently with little evidence of chest discomfort. According to current NCEP guidelines, patients with diabetes and without prior CHD are now considered to be

CHD 'equivalents' with identical risk reduction targets. The evidence for this approach is the equal incidence rates of MI in subjects without diabetes and with previous MI and in patients with diabetes and without previous MI. In a study of 4,000 MI patients in Finland (15% with diabetes), it was found that the 28-day mortality was 14% in diabetic men and 9% in nondiabetic men. In diabetic and nondiabetic women, mortality was 22% and 8%, respectively. In one half of patients with diabetes who die within 1 year of a first cardiac event, death is sudden. With the rising prevalence of diabetes in the United States, these findings have assumed an increasing importance.

In treating type 2 diabetes, the physician must deal with insulin deficiency and insulin resistance. Insulin resistance leads to increased insulin levels, which could have adverse effects on blood pressure and the endothelium, as well as on lipid levels. Insulin resistance can be reduced by weight reduction, when appropriate, and exercise.

Hyperglycemia is controlled by insulin and several groups of oral hypoglycemic agents, including the α-glucosidases and thiazolidinediones (TZDs). The former reduce glucose absorption, and the latter increase tissue sensitivity to insulin. Metformin (Glucophage®), a biguanide, has been useful in decreasing microvascular disease events in overweight patients with diabetes. The sulfonylureas increase pancreatic β-cell insulin release.

In the HOPE trial, patients with diabetes and at least one other risk factor for cardiovascular disease who were treated with the ACE inhibitor ramipril (Altace®) had a significant reduction in cardiovascular death (37%), nonfatal MI (22%), stroke (33%), and total mortality (24%) compared with a placebo group over a 4.5-year period. The use of ACE inhibitors also appears to decrease the development of albuminuria and overt nephropathy, as well as the development of diabetes, based on analysis of the HOPE study. Moreover, patients with diabetes treated with ACE inhibitors within 24 hours of MI in the GISSI-

3 trial had a reduced 6-week mortality (8.7% vs 12.4% treated conventionally).

Based on these considerations, it is recommended that the post-MI patient with diabetes receive aggressive control of blood sugar, with HbA_{1c} levels maintained at <7%. Metformin, among other agents, appears to have properties for risk reduction and should be used if there is no contraindication. High-fiber foods and foods with a low glycemic index should be emphasized, based on changes in blood sugar 3 hours after consumption of a reference food containing 50 g of available carbohydrate. The use of ACE inhibitors, beginning in the hospital period, is also strongly recommended.

Smoking

Health-care personnel recognize how difficult smoking cessation is for patients, although post-MI patients are more likely to stop than those with CHD who have not developed an acute coronary syndrome. However, smoking is the leading preventable cause of CAD and death in the industrialized world. There is compelling evidence that, in addition to adverse effects on platelet function and production of carboxyhemoglobin, the inhaled products of smoking, specifically nicotine, cause acute endothelial dysfunction. Cigarette smoking in general causes epicardial coronary artery constriction by stimulating coronary β-adrenergic receptors. Oxidative stress may mediate the effects on endothelial dysfunction caused by smoking, possibly associated with NO synthase inhibition.

Because there is no argument about the necessity of smoking cessation, especially after an MI, the challenge is how to achieve success. Perhaps the most comprehensive analysis of successful cessation interventions was accomplished by Kottke et al in 1988. They used a meta-analysis of 108 intervention comparisons in 39 controlled smoking cessation trials. The best results were achieved by multiple intervention techniques involving a team of physicians and nonphysicians. A combination of group and individual sessions had the greatest chance of success at 12 months. These trials used nicotine chewing gum extensively, but the nicotine patch had not yet been widely used. The meta-analysis found that, at 12 months, the average difference in quit rate between intervention and control groups was just under 6%, although there was considerable variation in individual programs, with the widest difference being 50%. Reinforcement and frequent contacts appear to increase successful compliance.

A study of a nurse-managed program concluded that such a program after MI was highly cost-effective in terms of lives saved, even if the program decreased the smoking rate by only 3/1,000 smokers (assuming a baseline of 26% smokers).

Considering the increasing encroachment on a physician's time by administrative duties and other responsibilities, it seems reasonable to try to develop comprehensive smoking cessation programs early in the post-MI period and, perhaps, extend the efforts through hospital-based contact after the patient has been discharged.

The best approach that an individual physician can take in dealing with a patient who persists in smoking is to: (1) provide a quit-smoking message with each patient contact, (2) attempt to set a quit-smoking date if the patient agrees, (3) reinforce this decision by telephone contact, and (4) provide group and individual health professional support through the following year, with the assistance of nicotine patches and bupropion if needed.

Gender Issues in Acute Myocardial Infarction

Substantial evidence indicates that women with acute MI are less aggressively managed than men. Information from the charts of 138,956 Medicare beneficiaries with acute MI in 1994 and 1995 indicated a decreased likelihood of interventional procedures in women of all age groups. Many of these differences were small, however, and early mortality was not affected. Further studies indi-

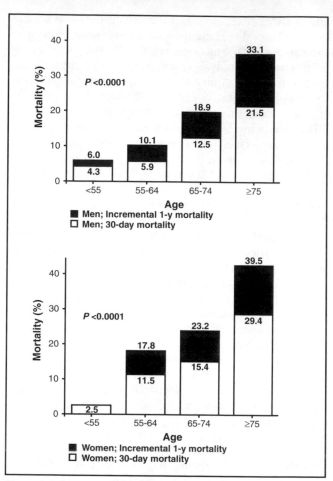

Figure 4-28: Sex differences in mortality after acute myocardial infarction in 2,867 consecutive patients from the Israeli Thrombolytic Survey Group Study. 30-day and 1-year crude mortality rates by age subgroups in (A) men and (B) women. *P* for trend <0.0001 for 30-day mortality and incremental 1-year mortality rates in both sexes. From Gottlieb et al, *Circulation* 2000;102:2484-2490, with permission.

cate that, in female MI patients who are older, have a greater prevalence of risk factors, and have a higher complication rate, there is no difference in aspirin use, β-blocker administration, or interventional procedures. In the Israeli Thrombolytic Survey Group Study, the 30-day mortality, but not the 1-year mortality, was higher for women (Figures 4-28 and 4-29). The difference in early outcome was explained by the older age of the women and greater co-morbidity. There is also evidence that women with angina are less likely to undergo diagnostic cardiac catheterization. This is especially salient because women experience chest pain as a symptom of CAD more frequently than men. One possible explanation for the discrepancy in diagnostic catheterization is the greater likelihood of normal epicardial coronary arteries in women with chest pain. Finally, stress test specificities tend to be lower in women than men (more false-positive tests). In terms of response to acute interventions, there have been concerns about a higher incidence of coronary reocclusion or complications after post-MI interventions. However, an evaluation of coronary patency rates of the infarct-related artery after thrombolysis indicated no significant gender difference at 90 minutes and at 5 to 7 days after the intervention.

Although women are less likely to have MI as the initial presentation of CAD, they have a higher fatality rate. Whether this is due to more atypical presentations in women or to the lower likelihood of women to seek medical attention for these symptoms is unclear. Biennial evaluation of the Framingham population, allowing for retrospective evaluation of MI incidence, found that unrecognized MI occurred in 38% of women compared with 28% of men. However, a recent report from the Heart and Estrogen/Progestin Replacement Study (HERS) of 2,763 postmenopausal women with CAD found that only 4.3% of women with nonfatal MI were unrecognized, based on serial electrocardiograms (ECG) and hospitalization information.

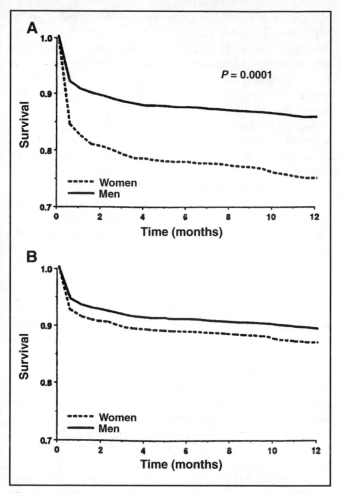

Figure 4-29: Survival in men and women at 12 months in the Israeli Thrombolytic Survey Group Study. (A) Unadjusted Kaplan-Meier curves, $P = 0.0001$ (log-rank test) for sex differences. (B) Adjusted survival curves predicted from Cox model. From Gottlieb et al, *Circulation* 2000;102:2484-2490, with permission.

An analysis of 384,878 patients enrolled in the US National Registry of Myocardial Infarction 2 between 1994 and 1998 showed a higher mortality in hospitalized women than in men (16.7% vs 11.5%). Younger women (<50 years) were more likely to die in the hospital than men of similar age (Figure 4-30). This difference decreased with age, and mortality rates were similar after age 74. After accounting for differences in medical history, severity of the MI, and management, risk was still higher in younger women. Indeed, after adjustment for these factors, one third of the risk difference was still unexplained. Possible reasons for the higher in-hospital mortality for younger women may relate to the underlying pathophysiologic state, including clotting mechanisms and the type of plaque disruption.

In an analysis of 6,826 patients discharged after MI, 2-year mortality was higher in women than in men (29% vs 20%) (Figure 4-31). As with the hospitalization period in other studies, only younger women had a higher posthospitalization mortality than men of similar age, with the sex difference in mortality decreasing with increasing age. This relationship held after adjustment for demographic characteristics and medical history. Unfortunately, there was no information on smoking patterns after hospitalization or posthospital treatment and compliance, which could have affected outcomes.

In summary, (1) women with acute MI are older and have more comorbidities than men at presentation; (2) the differences in outcome that favored men in earlier studies are decreased by multivariate adjustments; and (3) complications in the acute MI period and in the immediate posthospitalization period are more common in women, including complications from interventions such as thrombolysis.

The issue of hormone replacement therapy (HRT) after MI is examined in Chapter 3. However, we should indicate, on the basis of studies to date, that initiation of HRT after MI is now contraindicated for secondary prevention and that continuation of previous HRT should be

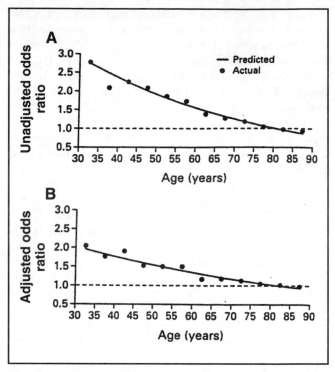

Figure 4-30: National Registry of Myocardial Infarction 2 (1994-1998). Odds ratio (women:men) for death during hospitalization for myocardial infarction, according to age. Risk ratio for women compared to men increased with decreasing age, reaching >2 at <35 years old. The unadjusted odds ratios (A) were derived from the model that included sex, age, the interaction between sex and age, and the year of discharge. The adjusted odds ratios (B) were derived from the model that included race, insurance status, medical history, severity of clinical abnormalities at admission, type of management in the first 24 hours after admission, and time of presentation. As seen in B, the adjusted odds ratios indicated a greater relative risk of mortality in women up to age 80. From Vaccarino et al, *N Engl J Med* 1999;341:217-225, with permission.

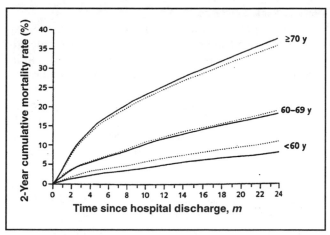

Figure 4-31: Sex-evaluated 2-year mortality data from 6,826 patients who survived hospitalization for acute myocardial infarction during ten 1-year periods between 1975 and 1995. Age-adjusted cumulative mortality rate from hospital discharge to 2 years in three age groups. Solid lines represent men; dotted lines represent women. From Vaccarino et al, *Ann Intern Med* 2001;134:173-181, with permission.

evaluated with caution. More generally, after the hospital period following MI, women should receive the same pharmacologic and lifestyle interventions as men, including aspirin, β-blockers, and ACE inhibitors. If anything, strict diabetic control should be more aggressively pursued in women. Because there is evidence that the 30-day postinfarction mortality is higher in women, every effort should be made to provide objective postdischarge evidence for myocardial vulnerability to ischemia by means of stress testing before discharge. The results of the Women's Health Initiative Primary Prevention Trial, which show an increase in cardiovascular events in the HRT group, strongly indicate a need for reconsideration of the efficacy of such interventions in regard to cardiovascular risk modification in general.

Novel Risk Factors

Aside from the standard risk factors, evidence suggests that other defined laboratory values, pathophysiologic processes, activity levels of endogenous substances, and infections may independently predict cardiovascular risk (Table 4-3).

Chylomicron remnants, triglycerides, and lipoprotein (a) [Lp(a)] have shown evidence for increased risk. The recently described 'metabolic syndrome,' which is associated with obesity and with small, dense LDL particles, decreased LDL-C, increased triglycerides, VLDL, decreased insulin sensitivity, and hypertension, may be reversed by appropriate lipid-lowering drugs and carbohydrate-modified diets with caloric restriction.

Lp(a), a particle that is structurally similar to LDL, competes with plasminogen for binding sites. Increased Lp(a) has been demonstrated in atheromatous plaques, and plasma levels have been increased in patients with CAD. The particle appears to be similar in activity to LDL-C in its propensity for increasing cholesterol accumulation in the arterial wall, enhancing foam cell formation, and generating free radicals in monocytes. The atherogenic potential of Lp(a) appears to be decreased by treatment of LDL-C. Niacin and a diet that emphasizes fish reduce Lp(a) levels. The clinical significance of Lp(a) reduction, independent of the effects on LDL-C reduction, remains to be determined.

Oxidative stress and triglycerides have been reviewed in the section on lipids. Homocysteine has been reviewed in the section on vitamins and antioxidants.

In addition to those mentioned above, there are many potential markers of risk for vascular occlusion, including fibrinogen, PAI-1, tPA mass, and von Willebrand factor antigen. Process markers of active vascular interactions that may indicate thrombosis or plaque breakdown include fibrin degradation products and D-dimer. Inflammatory markers that have been avidly assessed include

Table 4-3: Associations Between New and Established Risk Factors

Risk Factor	Association with Established Risk Factor
Left ventricular hypertrophy	Age, blood pressure, obesity
Homocysteine	Age, male, postmenopause
Hypertriglyceridemia	Diabetes, low HDL-C, small dense LDL-C, IDLP, obesity, smoking, postmenopause
Oxidative stress	Hypertriglyceridemia, smoking, hypertension, diabetes, low HDL-C, small dense LDL-C
Fibrinogen	Age, hypertension, diabetes, hypertriglyceridemia, LDL-C, low HDL-C, obesity, smoking, family history of premature CHD

HDL-C = high-density-lipoprotein cholesterol; LDL-C = low-density-lipoprotein cholesterol; IDLP = intermediate-density lipoprotein; CHD = coronary heart disease.

Adapted from Harjai et al, *Ann Intern Med* 1999;131:376-386, with permission.

high-sensitivity C-reactive protein (CRP), serum amyloid A (SAA), interleukins, and vascular and cellular fibrinogen adhesion molecules. An evaluation of selected risk factors from the Physicians' Health Study, which assessed the risk for MI in healthy middle-aged men, demonstrated that a combination of high-sensitivity CRP and a TC/HDL-C ratio was the best predictor of future MI, among choices that included high-sensitivity CRP, TC/HDL-C, tPA antigen, fibrinogen, TC, total homocysteine, and Lp(a), in order of predictability (Figure 4-32).

Infectious processes that are commonly thought to increase the risk for CHD include *Chlamydia pneumoniae*, *Helicobacter pylori*, and cytomegalovirus.

Inflammation and Infection

Inflammatory infiltrates have evoked considerable interest and investigation. These infiltrates have been found in MI and unstable angina plaques and associated with activated circulating neutrophils, lymphocytes, monocytes, and increased levels of inflammatory cytokines, as well as acute phase reactants such as CRP and SAA. Inflammation has been considered a contributor to the atheromatous process since the time of Virchow. Most recently, more clear-cut assessments of the biochemical nature of inflammation have focused on several major components of the inflammatory response. The components of greatest interest are CRP and SAA. Standards for the assessment of high-sensitivity CRP have helped to elucidate its effects on risk and allow replicative studies.

CRP levels have been correlated with low-grade inflammation and have been able to predict risk of first MI in apparently healthy men. A case-control study of patients with prior MI who subsequently developed recurrent MI or a fatal coronary event vs those with prior MI who remained free of subsequent events determined that those who developed subsequent events had the most consistently increased levels of CRP or SAA. Moreover, the risk of recurrent coronary events was independent of classic risk factors, such as smoking and lipid values. The elevated levels of both CRP and SAA may reflect a chronic inflammatory response, rather than a direct effect of either protein. In the CARE trial, a comparison of the groups with inflammation (CRP and SAA in 90th percentile) vs those without inflammation indicated that patients receiving the study drug (pravastatin) had a relatively lower risk for coronary events (Figure 4-33). In this regard, it is possible that statins may

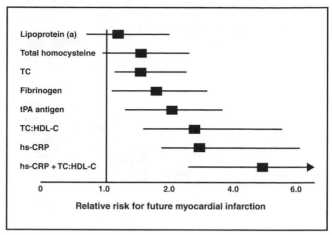

Figure 4-32: Physicians' Health Study. Relative risk for future myocardial infarction among apparently healthy middle-aged men according to baseline levels of some novel risk factors compared with total cholesterol (TC) and TC/high-density lipoprotein cholesterol (HDL-C) ratio. tPA = tissue plasminogen activator antigen; hs-CRP = high-sensitivity C-reactive protein. From Ridker, *Ann Intern Med* 1999;130:933-937, with permission.

have anti-inflammatory properties, independent of their effects on lipids (see Lipid Modification, this chapter).

Other effects of statins on modulation of the inflammatory process include inhibition of interactions between leukocyte antigens and intercellular adhesion molecules, independent of HMG-CoA reductase activity. However, there is evidence that HMG reductase, inhibited by statins, regulates the salient functions used by activated monocytes to invade endothelium. Aspirin has also been shown to reduce cardiovascular risk in direct relation to baseline levels of CRP.

Other studies of statin use have demonstrated beneficial effects on risk related to baseline CRP levels. For example, a prospective cohort of 985 patients with angiographically

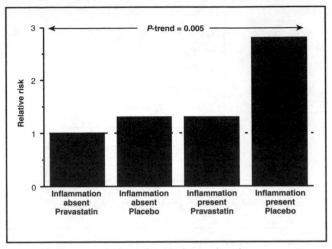

Figure 4-33: Results from the Cholesterol and Recurrent Events (CARE) trial. Relative risks of recurrent coronary events among postmyocardial infarction patients according to presence (both C-reactive protein [CRP] and serum amyloid A [SAA] levels ≥90th percentile) or absence (both CRP and SAA levels <90th percentile) of evidence of inflammation and by randomized pravastatin assignment. With inflammation present or absent, the relative risk for an event decreased in the pravastatin groups. From Ridker et al, *Circulation* 1998;98:839-844, with permission.

severe CAD had baseline lipid and CRP levels drawn and were followed for an average of 3 years. Although lipid levels at baseline were not predictive of survival, initiation of statin therapy predicted survival and was correlated with initial CRP levels (Figure 4-34 and Table 4-4). Another study of survivors of acute MI demonstrated that CRP levels tended to increase in patients on standard therapy and decreased in patients assigned to statin therapy, regardless of lipid level reached (Figure 4-35). These results support the evidence that the nonlipid effects of statins may include modulation of the inflammatory process and, thereby, may

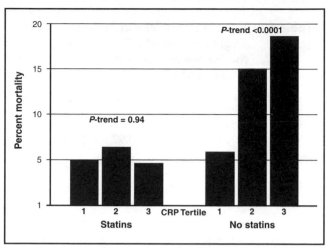

Figure 4-34: Effects of statins on mortality in patients with angiographically severe coronary artery disease stratified by tertiles of C-reactive protein (CRP) levels at baseline. For patients receiving statins, the risk due to increasing CRP was eliminated. For those not prescribed statins, a significant trend toward higher mortality existed along increasing CRP tertiles. From Horne et al, *J Am Coll Cardiol* 2000;36:1774-1780, with permission.

reduce cardiovascular risk. These data support the early use of statins after an acute coronary event, independent of lipid levels, based on possible plaque stabilization from the modulation of the inflammatory process.

Infectious agents have been suspected of playing a role in the development of atherosclerosis. Animal studies since the 1970s have provided evidence that viral agents such as herpesvirus and cytomegalovirus contribute to the pathogenesis of atherosclerosis. Much attention has also focused on bacterial agents, particularly *C pneumoniae* and *H pylori*. These organisms have been found in atheromatous plaques, especially *C pneumoniae*. Standard cardiovascular risk factors, CRP, advanced atherosclerosis, and

Table 4-4: Final Multiple Variable Cox Regression Model Showing the Independent Protective Effect of Statins

Risk Factor (n = 889)	Hazard Ratio
Age	1.08 per year
LVEF	0.97 per % increase
CRP	1.6 per tertile
Diabetes	1.7
Statins	0.49

CI = confidence interval; CRP = C-reactive protein; LVEF = left ventricular ejection fraction

Lipid levels, including total cholesterol, low-density lipoprotein cholesterol, and high-density lipoprotein cholesterol, were not predictive of long-term death in this model.

long-term cardiovascular mortality have correlated with antibodies against *Chlamydia*, *Helicobacter*, cytomegalovirus, and herpes simplex virus when adjusted for demographic factors. In response to the evidence of possible infectious etiologies of atherosclerosis, the results of secondary prevention trials using antibiotics in atherosclerosis are now being reported. Thus far, no reduction in cardiovascular events has been associated with antibiotic therapy (Figure 4-36). Two large-scale trials of more than 3,500 CHD subjects are under way. The Weekly Intervention With Zithromax for Atherosclerosis and Related Disorders (WIZARD) study evaluates 3 months of treatment. The Azithromycin Coronary Events Study (ACES) is a 1-year treatment study with 4 years of observation.

95% CI	P Value
1.05, 1.10	<0.0001
0.96, 0.99	<0.0001
1.3, 2.1	0.0002
1.1, 2.6	0.02
0.24, 0.97	0.04

Adapted from Horne, *Am Coll Cardiol* 2000;36:1774-1780, with permission.

These studies should be powerful enough to determine the significance of treatment of *C pneumoniae* infection as risk reduction for recurrent coronary events.

Fibrinogen

In pathophysiologic terms, the activation of fibrinogen can propagate arterial plaque and promote thrombosis by increasing platelet aggregation, increasing blood viscosity, stimulating smooth muscle cell migration, and, in the form of fibrin, binding with lipoprotein in the arterial wall. Fibrinogen levels are associated with recurrent ischemic events and angiographic severity of disease in patients with CHD. Population studies have clearly demonstrated the graded risk (Figure 4-37). In acute coronary syndromes, the risk for morbidity and mortality rise with increasing

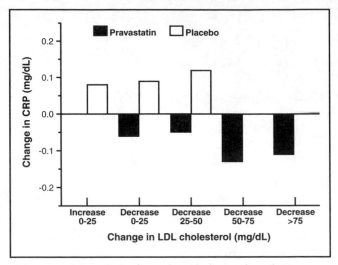

Figure 4-35: Results from the Cholesterol and Recurrent Events (CARE) trial. Mean change in C-reactive protein (CRP) levels over time according to observed changes in low-density lipoprotein cholesterol (LDL-C). Data are shown for those allocated to pravastatin (solid bars) or to placebo (open bars). A decrease in CRP was found in all subgroups assigned to pravastatin, and an increase in CRP was found in all groups assigned to placebo; these changes were unrelated to changes in LDL-C. From Ridker et al, *Circulation* 1999; 100:230-235, with permission.

fibrinogen levels. Numerous factors affect fibrinogen levels. Women and the elderly are more likely to have higher levels. Metabolic and environmental factors associated with fibrinogen levels include LDL-C and triglyceride levels, smoking, sedentary lifestyle, family history of premature CHD, hypertension, and diabetes. There is also evidence that socioeconomic factors associated with stress or job dissatisfaction, as well as with social environment and educational level, correlate with fibrinogen levels.

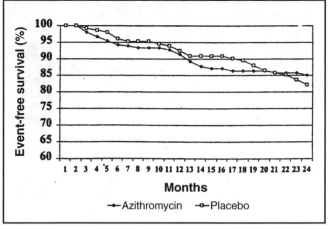

Figure 4-36: Coronary artery disease patients seropositive for *Chlamydia pneumoniae*. Kaplan-Meier primary event-free survival curves during 2 years of follow-up for patients randomized to azithromycin or placebo. No significant differences are seen. From Muhlestein et al, *Circulation* 2000;102:1755-1760, with permission.

Fibrinogen levels may be decreased by elimination of the factors associated with increased levels. Thus, smoking cessation, physical activity, weight loss, and decreased LDL-C and triglyceride levels decrease fibrinogen. Ticlopidine (Ticlid®) and especially the fibrates (Atromid-S®, Lopid®, Tricor®) have been associated with significant decreases in fibrinogen. Administration of bezafibrate in patients with CHD and high levels of fibrinogen has been shown in one study to decrease cardiac death and ischemic stroke.

Although the relationship of fibrinogen levels to cardiovascular risk has been recognized for several years, the assay and modification of fibrinogen levels in CHD have not been routine for several reasons, including lack of assay standardization, variation in levels in individual patients, and the tenuousness of evidence that decreases in fibrinogen

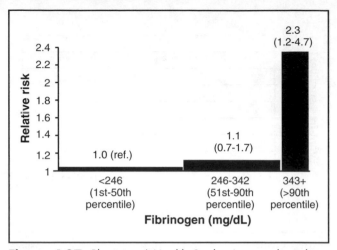

Figure 4-37: Physicians' Health Study. Age- and smoking-adjusted relative risk (95% confidence interval) of future myocardial infarction associated with baseline plasma fibrinogen levels. Numbers of cases/control subjects were 89/99 in the 1st to 50th percentiles, 73/80 in the 51st to 90th percentiles, and 37/20 in the >90th percentiles. From Ma et al, *J Am Coll Cardiol* 1999;33:1347-1352, with permission.

levels significantly lower risk for coronary events. However, there is now enough evidence to indicate that a high level of fibrinogen should be taken into account when assessing risk for coronary events.

Plasminogen Activator Mass

Just as fibrinogen may represent a process leading to coagulation, abnormalities of the fibrinolytic system perpetuate this potentially adverse effect on cardiovascular disease. Thus, there is increasing interest in evaluating the effects on fibrinolysis and its implications for cardiovascular risk. The leading candidates of interest are tPA and PAI-1. In the few studies evaluated, evidence suggests the correlation of PAI-1 levels with subsequent infarction in young survivors of MI. In patients with angina and angiographically verified CAD, increased plasma mass concentration of tPA, but not PAI-1, was related to 7-year mortality. Although it may seem paradoxical that tPA, which should be protective and whose activity is lowered by PAI-1, should be considered a risk factor, the increase in tPA mass reflects a decrease in tPA activity, a parallel to increased insulin levels when insulin sensitivity decreases.

One can reasonably speculate that the interplay of the fibrinolytic system elements is involved in ongoing events of coagulation developing from and leading to plaque disruption. Research on these elements suggests that there are reflectors of long-term risk (eg, hypertension, lipid levels) that may initiate processes leading to coronary events and that other reflectors of ongoing unstable pathophysiologic processes may represent ongoing plaque development and disruption (eg, fibrinolytic activators, fibrinogen and products, D-dimer). Consequently, it is conceivable that, in the future, long-term risk may be best assessed by the classic predictors but that, in acute coronary syndromes, the reflectors of ongoing processes, including the markers of inflammation, may provide greater predictors of short-term risk than those now routinely used.

Platelet Polymorphisms

As with other coagulation factors, platelets have a strong role in the active processes of plaque generation and disruption, leading to acute coronary events. Genetic predisposition to differences in platelet function, therefore, is important. Polymorphisms of interest include platelet glycoproteins involved in primary hemostasis, such as the von Willebrand factor receptor that forms the initial adhesion of the platelet to endothelium, the IIb/IIIa fibrinogen receptor required for platelet aggregation, and the PI^{A2} collagen receptor that stabilizes platelet adhesion. Recent evidence suggests a relation of such polymorphisms to acute coronary syndromes and complications after percutaneous coronary interventions. Considering the general

Table 4-5: Summary of 2001 ACC/AHA Guidelines for Prevention of Coronary Events in Patients With Established Cardiovascular Disease

Goals	Intervention Recommendations

Smoking:
  Goal
  Complete
  cessation
	Assess tobacco use. Strongly encourage patient and family to stop smoking and to avoid secondhand smoke. Provide counseling; pharmacologic therapy, including nicotine replacement and bupropion (Zyban®); and formal smoking cessation programs as appropriate.

BP control:
  Goal
  <140/90 mm Hg
  or <130/85
  mm Hg if heart
  failure or renal
  insufficiency;
  <130/80 mm Hg
  if diabetic
	Initiate lifestyle modification (weight control, physical activity, alcohol moderation, moderate sodium restriction, and emphasis on fruits, vegetables, and low-fat dairy products) in all patients with blood pressure ≥130 mm Hg systolic or 80 mm Hg diastolic. Add blood pressure medication individualized to other patient requirements and characteristics (ie, age, race, need for drugs with specific benefits) if blood pressure is not <140 mm Hg systolic or 90 mm Hg diastolic or if blood pressure is not <130 mm Hg systolic or 85 mm Hg diastolic for patients with heart failure or renal insufficiency (<80 mm Hg diastolic for patients with diabetes).

Goals

Lipid management:
  Primary goal
  LDL <100
  mg/dL

Intervention Recommendations

Start dietary therapy in all patients (<7% saturated fat and <200 mg/d cholesterol), and promote physical activity and weight management. Encourage increased consumption of ω-3 fatty acids. Assess fasting lipid profile in all patients and within 24 hr of hospitalization for those with an acute event. If patients are hospitalized, consider adding drug therapy on discharge. Add drug therapy according to the following guide:

LDL <100 mg/dL (baseline or on-treatment): Further LDL-lowering therapy is not required. Consider fibrate or niacin (if low HDL or high TG).

LDL 100-129 mg/dL (baseline or on-treatment): Therapeutic options: Intensify LDL-lowering therapy (statin or resin*). Fibrate or niacin if low HDL or high TG. Consider combined drug therapy (statin + fibrate or niacin) if low HDL or high TG.

(continued on next page)

Table 4-5: Summary of 2001 ACC/AHA Guidelines for Prevention of Coronary Events in Patients With Established Cardiovascular Disease *(continued)*

Goals	Intervention Recommendations
Lipid management: *(continued)*	LDL ≥130 mg/dL (baseline or on-treatment): Intensify LDL-lowering therapy (statin or resin*). Add or increase drug therapy with lifestyle therapies.
Lipid management: <u>Secondary goal</u> If TG ≥200 mg/dL, then non-HDL[†] should be <130 mg/dL	If TG ≥150 mg/dL or HDL <40 mg/dL: Emphasize weight management and physical activity. Advise smoking cessation. If TG 200-499 mg/dL: Consider fibrate or niacin *after* LDL-lowering therapy.* If TG ≥500 mg/dL: Consider fibrate or niacin *before* LDL-lowering therapy.* Consider ω-3 fatty acids as adjunct for high TG.
Physical activity: <u>Minimum goal</u> 30 minutes 3 to 4 days per week <u>Optimal</u> Daily	Assess risk, preferably with exercise test, to guide prescription. Encourage minimum of 30 to 60 minutes of activity, preferably daily, or at least 3 or 4 times weekly (walking, jogging, cycling, or other aerobic activity)

Goals	Intervention Recommendations
Physical activity: *(continued)*	supplemented by an increase in daily lifestyle activities (eg, walking breaks at work, gardening, household work). Advise medically supervised programs for moderate- to high-risk patients.
Weight management: <u>Goal</u> BMI 18.5-24.9 kg/m^2	Calculate BMI and measure waist circumference as part of evaluation. Monitor response of BMI and waist circumference to therapy. Start weight management and physical activity as appropriate. Desirable BMI range is 18.5-24.9 kg/m^2. When BMI ≥25 kg/m^2, goal for waist circumference is ≤40 inches in men and ≤35 inches in women.
Diabetes management: <u>Goal</u> HbA$_{1c}$ <7%	Appropriate hypoglycemic therapy to achieve near-normal fasting plasma glucose, as indicated by HbA$_{1c}$.

(continued on next page)

Table 4-5: Summary of 2001 ACC/AHA Guidelines for Prevention of Coronary Events in Patients With Established Cardiovascular Disease (continued)

Goals	Intervention Recommendations
Diabetes management: (continued)	Treatment of other risks (eg, physical activity; management of weight, blood pressure, and cholesterol).
Antiplatelet agents/ anticoagulants:	Start and continue indefinitely aspirin 75 to 325 mg/d if not contraindicated. Consider clopidogrel (Plavix®) 75 mg/d or warfarin (Coumadin®) if aspirin contraindicated. Manage warfarin to international normalized ratio = 2.0 to 3.0 in post-MI patients when clinically indicated or for those not able to take aspirin or clopidogrel.

BP = blood pressure; TG = triglycerides; BMI = body mass index; HbA_{lc} = major fraction of adult hemoglobin; MI = myocardial infarction; CHF = congestive heart failure; HDL = high-density lipoprotein; LDL = low-density lipoprotein.

* The use of resin is relatively contraindicated when TG >200 mg/dL.

Goals	Intervention Recommendations
ACE inhibitors:	Treat all patients indefinitely post-MI; start early in stable high-risk patients (anterior MI, previous MI, Killip class II [S_3 gallop, rales, radiographic CHF]). Consider chronic therapy for all other patients with coronary or other vascular disease unless contraindicated.
β-blockers:	Start in all post-MI and acute ischemic syndrome patients. Continue indefinitely. Observe usual contraindications. Use as needed to manage angina, rhythm, or blood pressure in all other patients.

† Non-HDL cholesterol = total cholesterol minus HDL cholesterol.

With permission from *J Am Coll Cardiology* 2001; 38:1581-1583.

Table 4-6: Specific Indications for Secondary Prevention After Hospital Discharge

Adapted from summary of 1999 ACC/AHA Guidelines for Management of Patients With Acute Myocardial Infarction and 2002 Updated Guidelines for Unstable Angina and Non-ST-Segment Elevation Myocardial Infarction

Classes: I: General agreement that treatment is beneficial, useful, and effective

IIa: Conflicting evidence for use; weight of evidence is in favor of efficacy

IIb: Conflicting evidence for use; efficacy is less well established

III: Evidence that treatment is not effective and in some cases may be harmful

Agent	Use	Class
ACE inhibitor	LVEF <40%, CHF, hypertension, diabetes	I
	Asymptomatic patients with LVEF 40% to 50%	IIa
	Normal or mildly abnormal LV function	IIb
β-blocker	All but low-risk patients	I
	Low-risk patients	IIa
	Survivors of non-ST-elevation MI	IIa
	Moderate or severe LV failure with close monitoring	IIb

Agent	Use	Class
Aspirin	All: 75-325 mg	I
	Clopidogrel (Plavix®) 75 mg/d when aspirin is not tolerated	I
	Aspirin and clopidogrel for 9 months	I
Lipid lowering	TLC diet (<30% fat calories, <7% saturated fat, <200 mg cholesterol)	I
Statin	Lipid-lowering agents with LDL-C >130 mg/dL	I
	Lipid-lowering agents with LDL-C >100 mg/dL	IIa
Fibrate/ Niacin	HDL-C <40 mg/dL and triglycerides >200 mg/dL	I
	Isolated HDL-C <40 mg/dL	IIa
Anticoagulants	Post-MI patients unable to take aspirin or equivalent	I
	Persistent atrial fibrillation or LV thrombus	I
	Extensive wall motion abnormalities	IIa
	Paroxysmal atrial fibrillation	IIa
	Severe LV dysfunction	IIb

(continued on next page)

Table 4-6: Specific Indications for Secondary Prevention After Hospital Discharge *(continued)*

Agent	Use	Class
HRT	Should not be given de novo Already taking HRT at time of MI: continue therapy	IIa
Calcium-channel blocker	Verapamil (Calan®, Covera®, Isoptin®, Verelan®) or diltiazem (Cardizem®, Cartia®, Dilacor®, Diltia®, Tiazac®) for ischemia if β-blockers are contraindicated	IIa
	Diltiazem in non-ST-segment elevation infarction without LV dysfunction, CHF, or pulmonary congestion	IIb
	Nifedipine (short acting) (Adalat®, Procardia®)	III
	Diltiazem and verapamil with LV dysfunction or CHF	III
Nitrates	Sublingual or spray nitroglycerin with instructions for use	

ACE = angiotensin-converting enzyme; LVEF = left ventricular ejection fraction; CHF = congestive heart failure; LV = left ventricular; MI = myocardial infarction; AHA = American Heart Association; LDL-C = low-density lipoprotein cholesterol; HDL-C = high-density lipoprotein cholesterol; HRT = hormone replacement therapy; TLC = Therapeutic Lifestyle Changes.
Note: Only 2002 recommendations are listed if they supersede 1999 recommendations.
Ryan et al, *Circulation* 1999;100:1016-1030;
Braunwald et al, *Circulation* 2002;106:1893-1900.

scope of cardiovascular risk after MI, it appears that future clinical trials should include such genetic predispositions, leading to a standardized assessment of susceptibility genes as part of a profile of short-term risk.

Conclusions

Risk factor modification for secondary prevention in post-MI patients should focus on the established, major, reversible factors. The 2001 ACC/AHA guidelines for prevention of recurrent coronary events in patients with cardiovascular disease provide recommendations and therapeutic targets for lipid management, blood pressure control, smoking cessation, physical activity, diabetes treatment, and weight control (Table 4-5). The ACC/AHA guidelines for the management of acute MI, based on the 1999 guidelines and the updated 2002 guidelines for unstable angina and non-ST-elevation MI, are summarized in Table 4-6. Of note in the revision is the recommended use of clopidogrel (Plavix®) when aspirin is contraindicated and the recommendation of fibrates or niacin when HDL-C levels are <40 mg/dL, especially when triglyceride levels are >200 mg/dL.

On the basis of the available recommendations, including NCEP ATP III, and continually accumulating data, we recommend that all post-MI patients receive dietary intervention (NCEP TLC diet or Mediterranean diet) and a statin if LDL-C is 100 mg/dL or greater. A fibrate or niacin should be considered when HDL-C is <40 mg/dL, especially with triglycerides >200 mg/dL, with the proviso that, in diabetic patients, adequate glucose control should be obtained and HDL-C and triglyceride levels reevaluated before considering this option. Therapy should be started at, or shortly after, hospital admission and continued for several months. At the conclusion of this time, the patient's total risk factor status should be reevaluated and treatment revised according to the 2001 ACC/AHA secondary prevention guidelines (Table 4-5). Based on the ACC/AHA 2000 guidelines for unstable angina and non-ST-elevation MI (the latest guideline on acute coronary syndromes), our recommendation for target blood pressure is <135/85 mm Hg after an acute coronary syndrome and <130/80 mm Hg if diabetes or chronic kidney disease is present. ACE inhibitors and aspirin should be given to all subjects, unless specifically contraindicated. We recommend β-blockers for all subjects unless specifically contraindicated.

Folate (1 to 5 mg) is advised for patients with homocysteine levels >15 mg/dL, preferably with vitamin B_6 and B_{12} supplementation. The role of other emerging risk factors remains investigational, and interest in them should not distract the clinician from intensive management of the established risk factors, which can achieve major reductions of cardiovascular mortality and morbidity in post-MI patients.

Suggested Readings

Amsterdam EA, Hyson D, Kappagoda CT: Nonpharmacologic therapy for coronary artery atherosclerosis: results of primary and secondary prevention trials. *Am Heart J* 1994;128:1344-1352.

Anderson JL, Muhlestein JB, Horne BD, et al: Plasma homocysteine predicts mortality independently of traditional risk factors and C-reactive protein in patients with angiographically defined coronary artery disease. *Circulation* 2000;102:1227-1232.

Anderson JW, Johnstone BM, Cook-Newell ME: Meta-analysis of the effects of soy protein intake on serum lipids. *N Engl J Med* 1995;333:276-282.

Ballantyne CM, Olsson AG, Cook TJ, et al: Influence of low high-density lipoprotein cholesterol and elevated triglyceride on coronary heart disease events and response to simvastatin therapy in 4S. *Circulation* 2001;104:3046-3051.

Braunwald E, Antman EM, Beasley JW, et al: ACC/AHA 2002 guideline update for the management of patients with unstable angina and non-ST-segment elevation myocardial infarction: a report of the American College of Cardiology/American Heart Association Task Force on Practice Guidelines (Committee on the Management of Patients With Unstable Angina). *J Am Coll Cardiol* 2002;40:1366-1374. Available at: http://www.acc.org/clinical/guidelines/unstable/unstable.pdf. Accessed on May 16, 2003.

Brown BG, Zhao XQ, Chait A, et al: Simvastatin and niacin, antioxidant vitamins, or the combination for the prevention of coronary disease. *N Engl J Med* 2001;345:1583-1592.

Chobanian AV, Bakris GL, Black HR, et al: The Seventh Report of the Joint National Committee on Prevention, Detection, Evaluation, and Treatment of High Blood Pressure. *JAMA* 2003;289:2560-2572.

De Lorgeril M, Salen P, Martin JL, et al: Effect of a Mediterranean type of diet on the rate of cardiovascular complications in patients with coronary artery disease. Insights into the cardioprotective effect of certain nutriments. *J Am Coll Cardiol* 1996;28:1103-1108.

Fonarow GC, French WJ, Parsons LS, et al: Use of lipid-lowering medications at discharge in patients with acute myocardial infarction: data from the National Registry of Myocardial Infarction 3. *Circulation* 2001;103:38-44.

Gottlieb S, Harpaz D, Shotan A, et al: Sex differences in management and outcome after acute myocardial infarction in the 1990s: A prospective observational community-based study. Israeli Thrombolytic Survey Group. *Circulation* 2000;102:2484-2490.

Harjai KJ: Potential new cardiovascular risk factors: left ventricular hypertrophy, homocysteine, lipoprotein(a), triglycerides, oxidative stress, and fibrinogen. *Ann Intern Med* 1999;131:376-386.

Horne BD, Muhlestein JB, Carlquist JF, et al: Statin therapy, lipid levels, C-reactive protein and the survival of patients with angiographically severe coronary artery disease. *J Am Coll Cardiol* 2000;36:1774-1780.

Kerzner B, Corbelli J, Sharp S, et al: Efficacy and safety of ezetimibe coadministered with lovastatin in primary hypercholesterolemia. *Am J Cardiol* 2003;91:418-424.

Lewis SJ, Moye LA, Sacks FM, et al: Effect of pravastatin on cardiovascular events in older patients with myocardial infarction and cholesterol levels in the average range. Results of the Cholesterol and Recurrent Events (CARE) trial. *Ann Intern Med* 1998;129:681-689.

Ma J, Hennekens CH, Ridker PM, et al: A prospective study of fibrinogen and risk of myocardial infarction in the Physicians' Health Study. *J Am Coll Cardiol* 1999;33:1347-1352.

Mikhaildis DP, Wierzbicki AS: The GREek Atorvastatin and Coronary-heart-disease Evaluation (GREACE) Study. *Curr Med Res Opin* 2002;18:215-219.

MRC/BHF Heart Protection Study of cholesterol lowering with simvastatin in 20,536 high-risk individuals: a randomised placebo-controlled trial. Heart Protection Study Collaborative Group. *Lancet* 2002;360:7-22.

Muhlestein JB, Anderson JL, Carlquist JF, et al: Randomized secondary prevention trial of azithromycin in patients with coronary artery disease: primary clinical results of the ACADEMIC study. *Circulation* 2000;102:1755-1760.

Prevention of cardiovascular events and death with pravastatin in patients with coronary heart disease and a broad range of initial cholesterol levels. The Long-Term Intervention with Pravastatin in Ischaemic Disease (LIPID) Study Group. *N Engl J Med* 1998; 339:1349-1357.

Randomised trial of cholesterol lowering in 4444 patients with coronary heart disease: the Scandinavian Simvastatin Survival Study (4S). *Lancet* 1994;344:1383-1389.

Ridker PM, Rifai N, Pfeffer MA, et al: Inflammation, pravastatin, and the risk of coronary events after myocardial infarction in patients with average cholesterol levels. Cholesterol and Recurrent Events (CARE) Investigators. *Circulation* 1998;98:839-844.

Ridker PM, Rifai N, Pfeffer MA, et al: Long-term effects of pravastatin on plasma concentration of C-reactive protein. The Cholesterol and Recurrent Events (CARE) Investigators. *Circulation* 1999;100: 230-235.

Ridker PM: Evaluating novel cardiovascular risk factors: can we better predict heart attacks? *Ann Intern Med* 1999;130:933-937.

Rossouw JE, Anderson GL, Prentice RL, et al: Risks and benefits of estrogen plus progestin in healthy postmenopausal women: principal results from the Women's Health Initiative randomized controlled trial. *JAMA* 2002;288:321-333.

Ryan TJ, Antman EM, Brooks NH, et al: 1999 update: ACC/AHA Guidelines for the Management of Patients With Acute Myocardial Infarction: Executive Summary and Recommendations: A report of the American College of Cardiology/American Heart Association Task Force on Practice Guidelines (Committee on Management of Acute Myocardial Infarction). *Circulation* 1999;100:1016-1030. Available at: http://www.acc.org. Accessed on May 16, 2003.

Sacks FM, Moye LA, Davis BR, et al: Relationship between plasma LDL concentrations during treatment with pravastatin and recurrent coronary events in the Cholesterol and Recurrent Events trial. *Circulation* 1998;97:1446-1452.

Sacks FM, Pfeffer MA, Moye LA, et al: The effect of pravastatin on coronary events after myocardial infarction in patients with average cholesterol levels. Cholesterol and Recurrent Events Trial investigators. *N Engl J Med* 1996;335:1001-1009.

Sacks FM, Tonkin AM, Shepherd J, et al: Effect of pravastatin on coronary disease events in subgroups defined by coronary risk factors: the Prospective Pravastatin Pooling Project. *Circulation* 2000;102:1893-1900.

Schnyder G, Roffi M, Pin R, et al: Decreased rate of coronary restenosis after lowering of plasma homocysteine levels. *N Engl J Med* 2001;345:1593-1600.

Schwartz GG, Olsson AG, Ezekowitz MD, et al: Effects of atorvastatin on early recurrent ischemic events in acute coronary syndromes: the MIRACL study: a randomized controlled trial. *JAMA* 2001;285:1711-1718.

Secondary prevention by raising HDL cholesterol and reducing triglycerides in patients with coronary artery disease: the Bezafibrate Infarction Prevention (BIP) study. *Circulation* 2000;102:21-27.

Smith SC Jr, Blair SN, Bonow RO, et al: AHA/ACC Guidelines for Preventing Heart Attack and Death in Patients With Atherosclerotic Cardiovascular Disease: 2001 update. A statement for healthcare professionals from the American Heart Association and the American College of Cardiology. *J Am Coll Cardiol* 2001;38:1581-1583.

Steinberg HO, Bayazeed B, Hook G, et al: Endothelial dysfunction is associated with cholesterol levels in the high normal range in humans. *Circulation* 1997;96:3287-3293.

Vaccarino V, Krumholz HM, Yarzebski J, et al: Sex differences in 2-year mortality after hospital discharge for myocardial infarction. *Ann Intern Med* 2001;134:173-181.

Vaccarino V, Parsons L, Every NR, et al: Sex-based differences in early mortality after myocardial infarction. National Registry of Myocardial Infarction 2 Participants. *N Engl J Med* 1999;341:217-225.

Vergnani L, Hatrik S, Ricci F, et al: Effect of native and oxidized low-density lipoprotein on endothelial nitric oxide and superoxide production: key role of L-arginine availability. *Circulation* 2000;101:1261-1266.

Chapter 5

Psychological Issues in Post-MI Patients

There is increasing evidence for the importance of psychosocial factors in the etiology of coronary heart disease (CHD). Behavioral characteristics and emotional stress are independent risk factors for both initial and recurrent coronary events. Psychosocial factors contribute to CHD on two major levels: (1) behavior-mediated physiologic alterations can affect multiple mechanisms that contribute to myocardial ischemia, atherothrombosis, and arrhythmogenesis, and (2) psychological adaptations to CHD influence compliance with medical management and lifestyle alteration to reduce the classic cardiac risk factors. Recent findings have confirmed the benefit of behavioral interventions on the course of patients with CHD, including those who have had an acute myocardial infarction (MI).

Despite the above findings, the psychosocial aspects of CHD remain underappreciated by most clinicians. This is probably because of our inability to apply to psychosocial function a simple method to measure cardiac risk and, thereby, determine a therapeutic target, as we can with the classic risk factors. The latter readily lend themselves to practical recommendations for management as embodied in the succinct American College of Cardiology (ACC) and American Heart Association (AHA) guidelines for secondary prevention of CHD (see Tables 4-5 and 4-6).

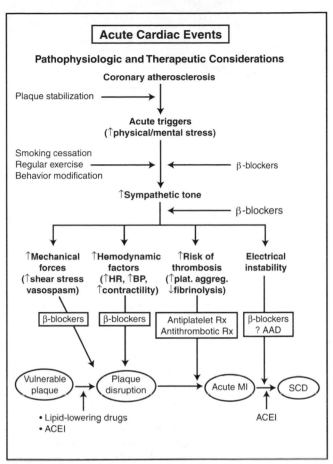

Figure 5-1: Interactions between chronic and acute risk factors influence pathophysiologic processes to modulate the likelihood that a patient with coronary heart disease will experience an acute event. Therapeutic influences act at several levels to modify the underlying risk. AAD = antiarrhythmic drug; ACEI = ACE inhibitors; SCD = sudden cardiac death. Figure developed initially by Deedwania P, MD. From Muller et al, *Circulation* 1997;96:3233-3239.

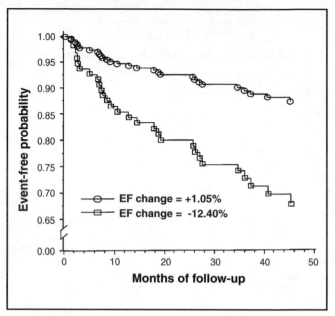

Figure 5-2: After performance of mental tasks during radionuclide ventriculography, patients were followed up over time (x axis). Probability of event-free survival is plotted as a function of mental stress-induced ejection fraction (EF) change plotted at two prototypical values, 1 standard deviation (SD) below (EF change = -12.40%) and 1 SD above (EF change = +1.05%) the mean of the entire sample (EF change = -6.73%). Curves are adjusted for baseline EF, history of myocardial infarction, and age. Relative risk associated with lower curve compared with higher curve is 2.40 (P = 0.024). With permission from Jiang et al, *JAMA* 1996; 275:1651-1656.

This chapter shows that basic patient assessment can reveal important information about a patient's psychosocial status and can suggest relevant interventions for overall management.

Psychosocial Factors

Five categories of psychosocial factors have been identified as contributing to the pathogenesis of CHD and recurrent coronary events after acute MI. They are personality factors and character traits, chronic life stress, anxiety, social isolation, and depression. These factors contribute to CHD by promoting adverse lifestyle choices (smoking, poor nutrition, inactivity) and by more direct physiologic mechanisms, such as neuroendocrine activation, altered hemodynamic function, and enhanced atherothrombosis. Management of patients in rehabilitation programs that include psychosocial intervention has been associated with improved psychological status and a decrease in recurrent CHD events.

Physiologic Effects of Psychosocial Stress

Direct Effects

The physiologic effects of emotional stress are mediated by the neuroendocrine system, hemostatic mechanisms, hemodynamic function, vascular reactivity, and control of cardiac rhythm. Acute stress may precipitate myocardial ischemia through stimulation of catecholamines, which can provoke myocardial ischemia and arrhythmias, impair endothelial function, and stimulate thrombogenesis. Some of these phenomena are depicted in Figure 5-1. Experimentally induced mental stress can impair coronary artery endothelial function, reduce coronary blood flow, and produce reversible myocardial perfusion defects in patients with coronary artery disease (CAD). Further clinical studies have shown that ischemia induced by mental stress in the laboratory setting predicts cardiac events in patients with CHD (Figure 5-2). Peripheral vascular reactivity is also modified, which possibly alters impedance to left ventricular stroke volume. These effects are mediated primarily through the sympathetic nervous system, although the renin-angiotensin system may also play a role. Arrhythmias can result from stress

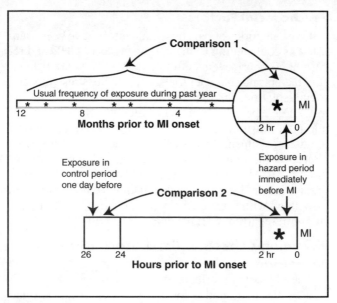

Figure 5-3: Schematic of the case-crossover study design to determine triggers of myocardial infarction (MI) on the basis of activity. The 2-hour period before MI onset is defined as the 'hazard period.' Comparison 1 contrasts exposure to potential triggering activities (such as episodes of anger or hostility) in the hazard period with the frequency of exposure expected, based on the reported usual frequency during the year before MI. In comparison 2, exposure in the hazard period is compared with exposure in a 'control period' at the same time on the preceding day. Together, the two methods of control information sampling permit assessment of recall and other biases inherent in the study of triggering. From Mittleman et al, *Circulation* 1995;92:1720-1725, with permission.

through catecholamine elevation, myocardial ischemia, and altered heart rate variability.

Specific physiologic effects of depression include increased cortisol activity, enhanced platelet reactivity, reduced heart rate variability, and impaired vagal control, all of which increase risk for further coronary events. Long-term effects of excess cortisol include elevated serum cholesterol and triglycerides, sodium retention, increased blood volume, reduced serum potassium, decreased ventricular ectopic thresholds, and increased sensitivity of arterioles to catecholamines. In turn, these changes can cause endothelial damage, produce lipid mobilization, activate macrophages, and induce arrhythmias. These pathophysiologic effects may also be provoked by emotions such as anxiety, hostility, and anger.

Effects on Risk Factors

Stress also interacts with the traditional risk factors. Stress can elevate total serum cholesterol, increase low-density lipoprotein cholesterol (LDL-C), and decrease high-density lipoprotein cholesterol (HDL-C). Both catecholamines and corticosteroids can decrease lipoprotein lipase activity, which lowers HDL-C. Patients with evidence of post-MI depression have poor adherence to risk-modifying behaviors and face increased mortality. In fact, the frequent failure of physicians, nurses, and patients to recognize depression in cardiac patients may prevent appropriate intervention. The decision to smoke may be a reaction to stress, but there appears to be better coping in patients who stop smoking. Overeating with consequent obesity is a maladaptive coping response to stress. Psychosocial and behavioral factors have also been linked to high blood pressure.

Effects of Psychological Factors on Coronary Heart Disease Events

Stress

In light of the profound physiologic effects of psychological function, it is not surprising that certain emotional and behavioral characteristics have been correlated with CHD events. The type A behavior pattern identified by Friedman and Rosenman almost 50 years ago, compared

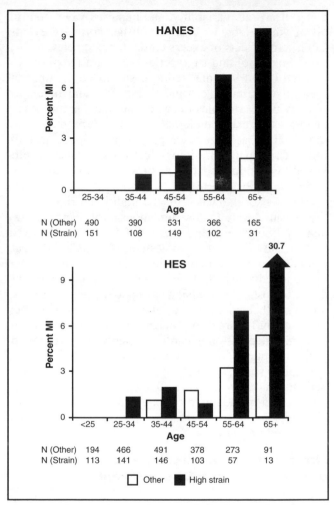

Figure 5-4: Prevalence of myocardial infarction by age and job strain in employed men, from the US Health and Nutrition Examination Survey (HANES) and the Health Examination Survey (HES). From Karasek et al, *Am J Public Health* 1988;78:910-918, with permission.

with the more placid type B personality, includes hostility, anger, competition, workaholism, impatience, and rapid speech. Some studies indicate that type A behavior confers a twofold risk of CHD and a fivefold risk of recurrent MI compared with type B behavior. However, other studies have shown no correlation between type A behavior and CHD risk. Confounding variables, such as social support, may explain some of these contradictory findings. In addition, it is possible that type A behavior may be associated with a willingness to modify lifestyle to decrease classic risk factors after a coronary event has occurred.

Acute, subacute, and chronic life stress may increase cardiovascular risk. The stress may result from bereavement, natural disasters, interpersonal relations, job-related concerns, or life changes. CHD has been related to these events in acute settings (Figure 5-3) and during prolonged exposure, especially in the work environment (Figure 5-4). Work-related stress, or 'job strain' as it has been termed in several models, has been associated with as much as a fourfold increase in risk for cardiovascular death. Worry, a form of anxiety, has been associated with more than a twofold increase in the risk of fatal CHD. In white men, worry appears to be associated with smoking, alcohol intake, and a family history of CHD.

Depression and Lack of Social Support

The prevalence of major depression is approximately three times higher in CHD patients than in the general population. Depression appears to result from coronary events and the increased risk for these events. The absence of social support, such as family, friends, and group and organizational activities, predicts increased cardiac risk. Several studies have shown a threefold increase in cardiac events and mortality in post-MI patients who have low levels of emotional support. Lack of social support is associated with high-risk behaviors, especially smoking and alcohol consumption.

Table 5-1: Psychosocial Interventions and Stress Management: Randomized Clinical Trial Efficacy for Reduction of CAD Events

Name	Year	# Patients
Ibrahim	1974	118
Rahe	1979	44
Fielding	1980	20
Stern	1983	64
Horlick	1984	116
Frasure-Smith	1985	457
Burgess	1987	180
Van Dixhoorn	1987	88
Guzetta	1989	80
Thompson	1990	60
Jones	1996	2,258

CAD events = myocardial infarction and cardiac death as well as, in some studies, unstable angina, congestive heart failure, and coronary bypass or angioplasty procedures

[†] P <0.05 vs controlled subjects

Intervention	Follow-up	CAD Events
Group psychotherapy	1 year	-65%[*]
Group therapy	4 years	-23%[*†]
Behavioral counseling and relaxation training	3 months	-10%
Group counseling	1 year	+24%
Education and group counseling	6 months	+133%
Nurse-managed environmental stress reduction/support	1 year	-51%[*†]
Cognitive behavior counseling and support	3 months	+20%
Relaxation exercises	2 to 3 years	-58%[†]
Music and relaxation response training	2 to 3 days	-100%[†]
Counseling	6 months	-57%
Psychological therapy, relaxation training, and stress management training	7 weeks	-9%

[*] These studies have demonstrated statistically significant cardiac mortality reduction associated with the intervention.

With permission from Bairey Merz et al, *Prev Cardiol* 1999;2:17-22.

Table 5-2: Comparative Efficacy of Interventions for Reduction of CAD Events

Intervention	CAD Risk Reduction (%)	# of Studies
Stress management	50[*†]	11
Lipid modification	33[*]	10
Aspirin	25[*]	65
β-blockers	20[*†]	31
Coronary artery bypass surgery	39[*†]	6

Recurrent CAD events = myocardial infarction and cardiac death as well as, in some studies, unstable angina and coronary bypass or angioplasty procedures

[*] These studies have demonstrated total mortality reduction associated with intervention.

[†] Preferential reduction of sudden cardiac death

With permission from Bairey Merz et al, *Prev Cardiol* 1999;2:17-22.

Behavioral Intervention After a Cardiovascular Event

According to a 1996 report of the US Department of Health and Human Services, adherence to cardiac rehabilitation services, including dietary changes, exercise, smoking cessation, and compliance with prescribed drugs, occurred in only 25% to 40% of patients after 6 months. This finding is of great concern because of the benefits that systematic rehabilitation programs have on prognosis in CHD. In this regard, controlled trials of psychosocial interventions in patients with CHD have demonstrated important reductions in cardiac events (Table 5-1). In addition, a comparative analysis of interventions in CHD patients revealed that stress management programs were at least as effective, or more effective, than medical and revascularization therapy in reducing CHD events (Table 5-2).

Intensive interventions to change behavior and, in turn, promote healthy lifestyles have emphasized frequent contact between the health professional and the patient as well as a decrease in the barriers to participation in treatment. These barriers include the physician's lack of reliance on behavioral approaches, perhaps due to lack of confidence that the patient will succeed. Additionally, physicians rarely promote patient self-efficacy, which depends on overcoming psychological obstacles. These obstacles, aside from the patient's lack of awareness about the importance of lifestyle changes, include post-MI depression, hostility, and anxiety. Consequently, coping with a patient's cognitive impairment and lack of understanding is essential.

Although the patient's partner is an integral part of the patient's social environment, there is inconsistent evidence that inclusion of the partner promotes behavioral change. Nonetheless, unmarried patients appear to be less likely to complete a cardiac rehabilitation program than those who are married. Certainly, the partner's behavior can also affect adherence to a treatment plan, especially if the partner smokes or prepares a high-fat diet.

Behavioral Approaches to Risk Factor Modification

In addition to behavioral issues related to the post-MI patient, the application of behavioral approaches to risk factor modification, including lifestyle changes, is critically important. Patients who continue to smoke must be willing to quit smoking before any effective intervention to stop smoking can be accomplished. This usually requires a 'quit smoking' message at every office visit. If the patient gives some indication that smoking cessation is desirable, the combined use of behavioral approaches may be successful. These approaches include enlisting the support of the patient's family, recommending group or individual sessions with a behaviorist or other health professional, and encouraging the patient to place cigarettes in inaccessible places or to be aware of situations in which cigarettes are routinely used. Written contracts and quit-smoking dates with early follow-up by the physician or another health professional may also be useful.

Stress monitoring and intervention programs that are managed by physicians or nurses after a patient's discharge from the hospital have been successful in modifying mortality rates (Tables 5-1 and 5-2). The most discouraging aspects of behavioral approaches are physicians' lack of knowledge about, or interest in, these activities or a misconception that these approaches do not usually work.

Approach to the Patient After an Acute Coronary Event

It is essential that physicians have a standardized approach to evaluating patients' behavioral and socioeconomic factors and understand what can be accomplished within the framework of psychosocial evaluation and how this can best be communicated to the patient. Physicians must also determine which health-care professionals can best support behavioral modification and how to bolster social support through the patient's family and/or friends. The first step in this process is a psychosocial profile of the patient that addresses issues such as family structure; home situation; job stress; economic status; evidence of anxiety, worry, depression, anger, or hostility; and activity status. Appropriate interventions may include individual or group counseling through a general cardiac rehabilitation program, stress modification sessions, and group sessions with other patients who have had comparable medical experiences, such as the Mended Hearts Clubs.

Even if elaborate behavioral modification sessions are unavailable because of the lack of a behaviorist, an office nurse or other staff member can assist in administering surveys specifically geared to determining anxiety status. These approaches may assist in directing the physician's goals of behavior modification.

The combination of lifestyle modification for reduction of classic risk factors with behavioral changes to assist in lifestyle modification would eventually provide an efficient way to improve the benefit of prevention programs. It is unlikely that the physician will be able to accomplish effective intervention alone if major anxiety, depression, or other psychological illnesses are present. Unfortunately, an untrained physician may not perceive evidence for such serious disorders unless he or she makes a determined effort to spend part of the office visit in attempting to identify the presence of these conditions.

Factors that play a role in compliance with lifestyle modification include the patient's perception of the threat of recurrent coronary events, of the physician, and of the therapeutic plan. Recommendations about behavior modification should have clear-cut goals, especially intermediate goals that can be readily achieved. Combination of verbal and written instructions is more effective than verbal alone. Ultimately, compliance depends on communication between the physician and the patient. Warmth and empathy are important attributes of the health care provider. The objective of providing the patient with clear-cut goals may be achieved by techniques such as emphasizing the importance of personal instruction, using short words and sentences, repeating instructions and documenting them in writing, asking the patient to repeat the instructions, and asking for the patient's negative feedback about instructions to prevent unforeseen obstacles.

Recognition of psychosocial risk affects patient compliance with drug therapy as well as lifestyle modifications to decrease classic risk factors. This can be best ac-

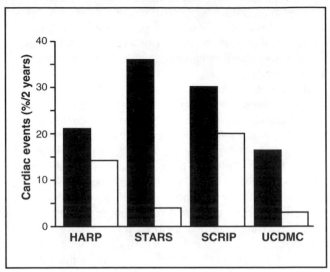

Figure 5-5: Two-year cardiac event rate in patients with cardiovascular disease in cardiac risk reduction programs. Dark bars = control patients, white bars = treated patients. HARP = Harvard Atherosclerosis Reversibility Project Study Group, SCRIP = Stanford Coronary Risk Intervention Project, STARS = St. Thomas Atherosclerosis Regression Study, UCDMC = UC Davis Medical Center (courtesy of Dr. C.T. Kappagoda).

complished by a systematic profiling of major psychosocial risk factors to accomplish an individualized treatment plan. Such a program can begin during hospitalization, with assessments of individual patient characteristics such as anxiety, depression, anger, worry, and socioeconomic evaluators. Job status is very important in this evaluation.

Many recent clinical trials have evaluated the potential utility of treating individual psychosocial factors. The Rush-Presbyterian-St. Lukes's Medical Center in Chicago has participated in the Enhancing Recovery in Coronary Heart Disease (ENRICHD) trial, in which more than 3,000 patients with major depression and/or social isolation were randomized to either a cognitive stress reduction program or usual care. Another relevant study, funded by the National Institutes of Health, is the Couples Intervention for Cardiac Risk Reduction Study, which was also conducted at Rush-Presbyterian-St. Luke's Medical Center. The latter study focuses on the evaluation of social interactions between patients who have had a cardiovascular event and their partners (spouse or live-in) to promote behavioral changes, such as improving adherence to a phase 2 rehabilitation program, weight loss program, and compliance with lipid-lowering medication. Other issues being studied include effects on patient mood, coping with illness, and quality of life. The University of California (Davis) Medical Center uses a traditional cardiac rehabilitation program as well as a more intensive Coronary Heart Disease Reversal Program. The latter involves the participation of spouses and includes vegetarian cooking, psychological support, and meditation sessions, in addition to exercise training and risk factor reduction. Results of this program (uncontrolled data) are shown in Figure 5-5 together with results of controlled trials. On the basis of these and similar programs, we recommend that a health professional hold a planning meeting with the patient and partner before hospital discharge to outline a comprehensive rehabilitation program to reduce psychological and other risk factors for further coronary events.

Summary

Psychosocial stress increases the occurrence of CHD events through its impact on the pathophysiology of CHD and its influence on patient compliance with medical therapy and lifestyle modification. Therefore, it is essential for physicians to be aware of the benefits of psychosocial intervention on recurrent events in the post-MI patient. The ability to identify patients with psychosocial stress and an awareness of basic strategies to reduce stress and depression are important to the success of the total rehabilitation effort to reduce recurrent CHD events. A systematic, personal approach tailored to the individual patient is the most effective method of reducing psychosocial stress and achieving the goal of optimal management of the post-MI patient.

Suggested Readings

Bairey Merz CN, Sabramanian R: Efficacy of psychosocial interventions and stress management for reduction of coronary artery disease events. *Prev Cardiol* 1999;2:17-22.

Braunwald E, Antman EM, Beasley JW, et al: ACC/AHA 2002 guideline update for the management of patients with unstable angina and non-ST-segment elevation myocardial infarction: a report of the American College of Cardiology/American Heart Association Task Force on Practice Guidelines (Committee on the Management of Patients With Unstable Angina). *J Am Coll Cardiol* 2002;40:1366-1374. Available at: http://www.acc.org/clinical/guidelines/unstable/unstable.pdf. Accessed on May 16, 2003.

Denollet J, Brutsaert DL: Reducing emotional stress improves prognosis in coronary heart disease. 9-year mortality in a clinical trial of rehabilitation. *Circulation* 2001;104:2018-2023.

Karasek RA, Theorell T, Schwartz JE, et al: Job characteristics in relation to the prevalence of myocardial infarction in the US Health Examination Survey (HES) and the Health and Nutrition Examination Survey (HANES). *Am J Public Health* 1988;78:910-918.

Mittleman MA, Maclure M, Sherwood JB, et al: Triggering of acute myocardial infarction onset by episodes of anger. Determinants of Myocardial Infarction Onset Study Investigators. *Circulation* 1995;92:1720-1725.

Muller JE, Kaufman PG, Luepker RV, et al: Mechanisms precipitating acute cardiac events: review and recommendations of an NHLBI workshop. National Heart, Lung, and Blood Institute. Mechanisms Precipitating Acute Cardiac Events Participants. *Circulation* 1997;96:3233-3239.

Rozanski A, Blumenthal JA, Kaplan J: Impact of psychological factors on the pathogenesis of cardiovascular disease and implications for therapy. *Circulation* 1999;99:2192-2217.

Ryan TJ, Antman EM, Brooks NH, et al: ACC/AHA guidelines for the management of patients with acute myocardial infarction:

1999 update: a report of the American College of Cardiology/ American Heart Association Task Force on Practice Guidelines (Committee on Management of Acute Myocardial Infarction). Available at: http://www.acc.org. Accessed on May 16, 2003.

Williams JE, Paton CC, Siegler IC, et al: Anger proneness predicts coronary heart disease risk: prospective analysis from the Atherosclerosis Risk in Communities (ARIC) study. *Circulation* 2000; 101:2034-2039.

Chapter 6

Convalescence: From Intensive Care to Full Activity

Two important aspects of contemporary care of patients with uncomplicated acute coronary syndromes (myocardial infarction [MI] or unstable angina) and low-risk features have been shortened hospital stay and relatively rapid return to full activity within the limitations imposed by the underlying coronary heart disease. Pathologic studies performed more than 60 years ago suggested that prolonged rest was required to promote healing of the infarcted myocardium. However, this concern has not been borne out by subsequent clinical experience. In fact, early resumption of limited activity, with gradual progression, has multiple beneficial physiologic and psychological effects in contrast to the deleterious influence of prolonged bedrest. Physical activity averts venous thrombosis, pulmonary emboli, loss of muscle strength, deconditioning of cardiovascular reflexes, impaired bowel and bladder function, and cardiac invalidism, and it significantly enhances patients' morale.

The salutary effect of bed-to-chair activity on limiting the development of venous thrombi in patients in a cardiac care unit (CCU) is shown in Table 6-1. Evidence of venous thrombi, as reflected by radioisotope fibrinogen labeling, was markedly reduced in patients managed with early ambulation compared to a matched control group. These findings were further confirmed by venography in selected patients.

Patients should have constant electrocardiographic monitoring from admission until discharge, and physical activity should be reduced or curtailed upon any evidence of new signs or symptoms of myocardial ischemia, cardiac failure, or arrhythmias.

Hospital Phase

Modest activity can begin within 24 hours of admission to the CCU in appropriate patients, as indicated by clinical stability and absence of cardiac symptoms. Activity should comprise brief periods out of bed, such as at mealtime. It is easier for most patients to use a bedside commode than a bedpan for bowel movements, and this option should be available. In addition to electrocardiographic monitoring for ischemia and arrhythmias, heart rate and blood pressure should be measured to determine the effect of activities performed out of bed. By day 2, the patient can walk slowly in the room in preparation for transfer to a telemetry unit the following day. Passive range-of-motion exercises can be initiated 24 hours after admission in patients with uncomplicated coronary events. If these maneuvers do not induce signs or symptoms, the patient can be transferred after 48 hours to a unit with telemetric monitoring.

On the telemetry unit, the patient's supervised activity can progress to spending several hours each day out of bed, including meals, bathroom functions, and slow, unassisted walking (initially under supervision) in the room and beyond. Discharge can be planned when the patient seems able to perform the basic activities of daily living unassisted without signs or symptoms. At that time, a predischarge submaximal exercise test is usually performed.

Predischarge Exercise Test

This method affords important prognostic information (Chapter 2) and complements the clinical assessment with

Table 6-1: Results of Early Mobilization in Acute Myocardial Infarction

Group	Subjects (N)
A—Early mobilization	
Killip II	12
Killip III	9
B—Late mobilization	
Killip II	3
Killip III	5
Total	29

From Miller et al, *Ann Intern Med* 1976;84:700-703, with permission.

quantitative data on functional capacity and the threshold for any signs or symptoms. A submaximal test is usually performed; symptom-limited testing, if indicated, is reserved for 1 to 2 months after hospital discharge. A variety of end points have been used for submaximal testing, including 70% of maximum predicted heart rate, heart rate of 130 bpm, and two stages of the Bruce protocol. The activity level achieved during treadmill testing can be related to comparable occupational, recreational, and self-care functions, as shown in Table 6-2. The energy requirements of these activities are indicated in terms of metabolic equivalents, or METs (multiples of resting oxygen consumption). One MET equals 3.5 cc/kg/min, which is considered resting, or basal, energy expenditure. For example, the energy required for walking at a rate of 2.5 mph, dressing, or showering is 3 METs, or a threefold increase over resting energy requirements. Ability to safely achieve this level on

¹²⁸I-Fibrinogen Test		Venography	
Positive	Negative	Positive	Negative
0	12	0	4
2	7	1	3
1	2	1	2
4	1	4	1
7	22	6	10

an exercise test is helpful in considering the timing of discharge and the adequacy of medical therapy. An additional advantage of the exercise test is the positive effect a successful study has on the morale of the patient and his or her spouse and family.

The progression from CCU admission to discharge in patients with uncomplicated coronary events usually takes 3 to 5 days, depending on the response of the patient, the support system at home, and the clinical circumstances. Patients with an uncomplicated MI who have undergone reperfusion therapy by primary coronary angioplasty usually do not require predischarge exercise testing and can commonly be discharged as early as 3 days after admission. By contrast, an elderly patient with limited social support may require longer hospitalization before attaining sufficient evidence of physical independence and self-confidence necessary for discharge.

Table 6-2: Energy Requirements of Various Physical Activities

Intensity	Self-Care or Home
Very light <3 METs* (<10 mL/kg/min)	Washing, dressing Desk work, writing Washing dishes Driving automobile
Light 3-5 METs (11-18 mL/kg/min)	Cleaning windows Raking leaves Power lawn mower Carrying objects (15-30 lb)
Moderate 5-7 METs (18-25 mL/kg/min)	Garden work (light) Climbing stairs Carrying objects (30-60 lb)
Heavy 7-9 METs (25-32 mL/kg/min)	Sawing wood Heavy shoveling Stairs (moderate pace) Carrying objects (60-90 lb)

*1 MET = resting level of energy expenditure (3.5 cc/kg/min)

Any of the above activities can cause increased cardiac work if associated with psychological stress.

Posthospital Phase

Progressive activity gradually continues in the first 1 to 2 weeks after discharge. Depending on the individual circumstances, this progression comprises walking at a slow to medium pace for 5 to 10 minutes one or more

Occupational	Recreational
Sitting, clerical	Shuffleboard
Standing (store clerk)	Horseshoes
Driving truck	
Stocking shelves (light objects)	Dancing
Light carpentry	Golf (walking)
Auto repair	Sailing
	Horseback riding
	Volleyball
	Tennis (doubles)
Carpentry	Tennis (singles)
Shoveling dirt	Skiing
	Light backpacking
	Basketball
	Skating
Digging ditches	Canoeing
Pick and shovel	Mountain climbing

times daily, stair climbing once or twice daily, and similar functions (Table 6-2). If these activities are not associated with symptoms, their frequency, duration, and intensity can be gradually increased over the ensuing 2 to 3 weeks. During this period, the patient should have an outpatient visit to assess progress, receive guidelines for further activity, and evaluate the response to medications. Enrollment in a formal cardiac rehabilitation program can also be considered (Chapter 5). These programs confer multiple benefits, including a systematic approach to resumption of full activity within the limits of residual cardiac function, risk factor reduction, and psychologic support. Depending on the patient's occupation and physiologic status, return to part-time work is also considered at this time, with full-time return following according to patient-specific and job-related factors. A symptom-limited exercise test is useful at this time, especially if the occupational activity is more than moderate. Improvement in exercise tolerance increases progressively for 3 to 6 months, with the level reached depending on the patient's age, extent of infarction, comorbidity, and involvement in formal or informal rehabilitation activities. In the modern era, in which acute coronary reperfusion therapy is accomplished in many patients, return to full-time work can appropriately occur within 4 weeks after an uncomplicated MI, but it may take considerably longer, depending on the individual patient and occupation.

Sexual Activity

Although sexual activity is important to most patients and their partners, physicians and patients often neglect to discuss it. Many patients are reluctant to raise this sensitive issue, but physicians should include it in predischarge counseling. Classic studies have shown that the energy expenditure associated with sexual activity is approximately 5 METs. It has been equated to the effort of climbing two flights of stairs or exertion to a heart rate of 130 bpm and a systolic blood pressure of about 150 mm Hg. The latter hemodynamic variables may be exceeded in individual subjects. The increase in metabolic demand is relatively brief, with orgasm lasting 10 to 16 seconds, preceded by 5 minutes or more of stimulation, and a resolution phase of less than 20 seconds. Patients who have progressed to the equivalent of 5 METs of physical activity can appropriately resume sexual function. This is usually after 2 weeks at home but varies with individual circumstances. It has been further recommended that the partner without a recent cardiac event assume the more active role when sexual activity is resumed. When the male partner is recovering from an MI, this would be exemplified by practicing the Lilith position (woman above) for at least the initial period of sexual function.

Management of Erectile Dysfunction

Many factors can contribute to erectile dysfunction, some of which are prevalent in men who have had an MI, including the aging process, vascular disease, diabetes, sexual performance anxiety, and certain drugs. Among the latter are β-blockers, thiazides, and centrally-acting antihypertensives. Noncardiac drugs associated with erectile dysfunction include alcohol, cimetidine, and ketoconazole. Treatment of erectile dysfunction includes elimination of potentially responsible drugs, if possible, and appropriate referral for management of nonvascular disease (eg, endocrine, neurologic, or psychological disorders). Therapeutic options vary widely, ranging from pharmacologic to surgical (prosthesis) methods.

Sildenafil (Viagra®), the drug of choice for most men with erectile dysfunction, is also the most frequent treatment for this condition. By selective inhibition of phosphodiesterase type 5, sildenafil markedly increases cyclic GMP concentration in the penis, increasing smooth muscle relaxation and augmenting erection through enhanced blood engorgement. The drug has no effect on the penis when nitric oxide and cyclic GMP concentrations are low, as in the absence of sexual stimulation. Sildenafil has been evaluated in multiple clinical trials and has been associated with significantly improved sexual performance and satisfaction. Adverse events, which are dose-related, are

Table 6-3: Recommendations For Use of Sildenafil by Men With Cardiac Disease*

1. Sildenafil is absolutely contraindicated in men taking long-acting or short-acting nitrate drugs.

2. If the man has stable coronary disease and does not need nitrates regularly, the risks of sildenafil should be carefully discussed with him. If the man requires nitrates because of mild-to-moderate exercise limitation due to coronary disease, sildenafil should not be given.

3. All men taking an organic nitrate (including amyl nitrate) should be informed about the nitrate-sildenafil hypotensive interaction.

4. Men must be warned of the danger of taking sildenafil 24 hours before or after taking a nitrate preparation.

5. Before sildenafil is prescribed, treadmill testing may be indicated in some men with cardiac disease to assess the risk of cardiac ischemia during sexual intercourse.

6. Initial monitoring of blood pressure after the administration of sildenafil may be indicated in men with congestive heart failure who have borderline low blood pressure and low volume status and men being treated with complicated, multidrug antihypertensive regimens.

* Recommendations prepared by the American Heart Association.

mild to moderate and largely reflect vasodilation (headache, flushing, nasal congestion). The rate of serious cardiovascular events associated with sildenafil use is estimated to be very low. There have been 130 reported deaths in more than 3 million men receiving the drug. However, the combination of sildenafil with concurrent nitrate therapy has resulted in hypotension and death. Therefore, nitrate therapy is an absolute contraindication to the use of sildenafil. The guidelines of the American Heart Association for the use of sildenafil in men with cardiovascular disease are shown in Table 6-3.

Suggested Readings

Braunwald E, Antman EM, Beasley JW, et al: ACC/AHA 2002 guideline update for the management of patients with unstable angina and non-ST-segment elevation myocardial infarction: a report of the American College of Cardiology/American Heart Association Task Force on Practice Guidelines (Committee on the Management of Patients With Unstable Angina). *J Am Coll Cardiol* 2002;40:1366-1374. Available at: http://www.acc.org/clinical/guidelines/unstable/unstable.pdf. Accessed on May 16, 2003.

Cheitlin MD, Hutter AM Jr, Brindis RG, et al. Use of sildenafil (Viagra) in patients with cardiovascular disease. *Circulation* 1999;99:168-177. [Erratum, *Circulation* 1999;100:2389.]

Miller RR, Lies JE, Carretta RF, et al: Prevention of lower extremity venous thrombosis by early mobilization. Confirmation in patients with acute myocardial infarction by 125I-fibrinogen uptake and venography. *Ann Intern Med* 1976;84:700-703.

Ryan TJ, Antman EM, Brooks NH, et al: ACC/AHA guidelines for the management of patients with acute myocardial infarction: 1999 update: a report of the American College of Cardiology/American Heart Association Task Force on Practice Guidelines (Committee on Management of Acute Myocardial Infarction). Available at: http://www.acc.org. Accessed on May 16, 2003.

Guidelines Relevant to the Management of Patients Who Have Had Myocardial Infarction (or Other Acute Coronary Syndrome), 1996-2002

American Heart Association (AHA)– www.americanheart.org

- Summary of the Scientific Conference on the Efficacy of Hypocholesterolemic Dietary Interventions (December 1996)
- In-Hospital Resuscitation (April 1997)
- Fiber, Lipids, and Coronary Heart Disease (June 1997)
- Aspirin as a Therapeutic Agent in Cardiovascular Disease (October 1997)
- Very Low Fat Diets (September 1998)
- Obesity: Impact on Cardiovascular Disease (October 1998)
- AHA Science Advisory: Homocyst(e)ine, Diet, and Cardiovascular Diseases (January 1999)
- American College of Cardiology (ACC)/AHA Expert Consensus Document: Use of Sildenafil (Viagra®) in Patients With Cardiovascular Disease (January 1999)

- ACC/AHA Guidelines for the Management of Patients With Acute Myocardial Infarction (August 1999)
- ACC/AHA Guidelines for Coronary Artery Bypass Graft Surgery (September 1999)
- AHA/American Association of Cardiovascular and Pulmonary Rehabilitation (AACVPR) Scientific Statement: Core Components of Cardiac Rehabilitation/Secondary Prevention Programs (August 2000)
- An Eating Plan for Healthy Americans: Our American Heart Association Diet (October 2000)
- AHA Science Advisory: Stanol/Sterol Ester Containing Foods and Blood Cholesterol Levels (February 2001)
- Summary of the Scientific Conference on Dietary Fatty Acids and Cardiovascular Health (February 2001)
- AHA Science Advisory: Lyon Diet Heart Study: Benefits of a Mediterranean-Style, National Cholesterol Education Program (NCEP)/AHA Step I Dietary Pattern on Cardiovascular Disease (April 2001)
- NCEP: Third Report of the Expert Panel on Detection, Evaluation, and Treatment of High Blood Cholesterol in Adults (Adult Treatment Panel III) (May 2001)
- Guide to Anticoagulant Therapy: Heparin (June 2001)
- ACC/AHA Guidelines to Percutaneous Coronary Intervention (June 2001)
- Hormone Replacement Therapy and Cardiovascular Disease (July 2001)
- ACC/AHA/European Society of Cardiology (ESC) Guidelines for the Management of Patients With Atrial Fibrillation (August 2001)
- AHA/ACC Guidelines for Preventing Heart Attack and Death in Patients With Atherosclerotic Cardiovascular Disease: 2001 Update (September 2001)
- Renal Considerations in Angiotensin Converting Enzyme Therapy (October 2001)

- ACC/AHA Guidelines for the Evaluation and Management of Chronic Heart Failure in the Adult (November 2001)
- ACC/AHA Guideline Update for Perioperative Cardiovascular Evaluation for Noncardiac Surgery (January 2002)
- Secondary Prevention of Coronary Heart Disease in the Elderly (With Emphasis on Patients ≥75 Years of Age) (April 2002)
- Prevention Conference VI: Diabetes and Cardiovascular Disease (May 2002)
- ACC/AHA/National Heart, Lung, and Blood Institute (NHLBI) Clinical Advisory on the Use and Safety of Statins (June 2002)
- ACC/AHA 2002 Guideline Update for Exercise Testing (September 2002)
- ACC/AHA/North American Society of Pacing and Electrophysiology (NASPE) 2002 Guideline Update for Implantation of Cardiac Pacemakers and Antiarrhythmia Devices (September 2002)
- ACC/AHA Guideline Update 2002 for the Management of Patients With Unstable Angina and Non-ST-Segment Elevation Myocardial Infarction (October 2002)
- Fish Consumption, Fish Oil, ω-3 Fatty Acids, and Cardiovascular Disease (November 2002)
- ACC/AHA 2002 Guideline Update for the Management of Patients With Chronic Stable Angina (November 2002)

National Heart, Lung, and Blood Institute (NHLBI)–www.nhlbi.nih.gov

- The Seventh Report of the Joint National Committee on the Prevention, Detection, Evaluation and Treatment of High Blood Pressure (May 2003)

American College of Physicians-American Society of Internal Medicine (ACP-ASIM)– www.acponline.org

- Risk Stratification After Myocardial Infarction. *Ann Intern Med* 1997;126:556-582.
- Perioperative Assessment and Management of Risk From Coronary Artery Disease. *Ann Intern Med* 1997; 127:309-328.
- Guidelines for Management of Patients With Chronic Stable Angina. *J Am Coll Cardiol* 1999;33:2092-2197.

Canadian Cardiovascular Society (CCS)– www.ccs.ca

- Evaluation and Management of Chronic Ischemic Heart Disease (1997)
- Prevention of Sudden Death From Ventricular Arrhythmia (1999)
- Women and Ischemic Heart Disease (2000)
- Management of Heart Disease in the Elderly Patient (2002 [Draft])

European Society of Cardiology (ESC)– www.escardio.org

- Acute Myocardial Infarction: Pre-hospital and In-hospital Management (1996)
- The Pre-hospital Management of Acute Heart Attacks (1998)
- Management of Chest Pain (2002)
- Management of Acute Coronary Syndromes in Patients Presenting *Without* Persistent ST-segment Elevation (2002 [supersedes 2000 Guidelines])

Appendix B

Recommended Web Sites

- **ACCardio:** www.cardiosource.com
- **Cochrane Controlled Trials Register:**
  www.cochrane.org
- **EMBASE:** www.embase.com
- **Evidence-based Cardiovascular Medicine:**
  www.harcourt-international.com/journals/ebcm
- **Hurst's The Heart:**
  www.cardiology.accessmedicine.com
- **MEDLINE:** www.medlineplus.gov
- **TRIP:** www.tripdatabase.com

Appendix C

Recommended Books

1. Braunwald E, Zipes DP, Libby P, eds: *Heart Disease: A Textbook of Cardiovascular Medicine.* 6th ed. Philadelphia, WB Saunders, 2001.

2. Fuster V, Alexander RW, O'Rourke RA, et al, eds: *Hurst's The Heart.* New York, McGraw-Hill Medical Publishing Division, 2001.

3. Kloner RA, Birnbaum Y, eds: *Cardiovascular Trials Review.* 7th ed. Darien, CT, LeJacq Communications, 2002.

4. Topol EJ, ed: *Textbook of Cardiovascular Medicine.* 2nd ed. Philadelphia, Lippincott Williams & Wilkins, 2002.

Index